Step by Step

Art of
Endosuturing

Step by Step

Art of
Endosuturing

Parveen Bhatia

MS, FICS

Consultant Laparoscopic Surgeon & Medical Director,
Global Hospital & Endosurgery Institute, New Delhi

Suviraj J John

MS, DNB (Surgery), PGDH & HM

Consultant Laparoscopic Surgeon,
Bangalore Baptist Hospital, Bangalore

JP Singh Deed

MS, DNB, MNAMS, MRCS (Edin)

Consultant Laparoscopic Surgeon &
International Visiting Faculty for Laparoscopy,
Sant Parmanand Hospital, New Delhi

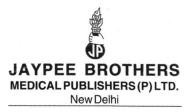

JAYPEE BROTHERS
MEDICAL PUBLISHERS (P) LTD.
New Delhi

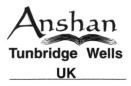

Anshan
Tunbridge Wells
UK

First published in the UK by

Anshan Ltd.
in 2006
6 Newlands Road
Tunbridge Wells
Kent TN4 9AT, UK

Tel/Fax: +44 (0)1892 557767
E-mail: info@anshan.co.uk
www.anshan.co.uk

ISBN-10 1 904798 829
ISBN-13 978 1 904798 82 8

British Library Cataloguing in Publication Data
A catalogue record for this book is available from the British Library

Printed in India by Paras Offset Pvt. Ltd., Naraina, New Delhi.

Foreword

Art of endoscopic suturing is the most important technique of laparoscopic surgery that elevates a basic laparoscopic surgeon to higher level where one can perform advanced laparoscopic surgeries. This extraordinary manual represents a successful effort to bring together all basic concepts and techniques of endosuturing in the current era of laparoscopic surgery. The authors have addressed the importance of endosuturing, its utility, difference between it and the conventional suturing and the difficulties in mastering art of endosuturing.

This book illustrates various types of knotting and suturing, its advantages and disadvantages, indications and methodology of applying these techniques. This book provides easy-to-follow, step-by-step detail for various types of endosuturing and knotting in text and in a collection of superb line drawings. These drawings are clear and easily followed and provide adequate information regarding the various procedures. This method of presentation greatly eases the learning process and will help the surgeons to master these techniques in a short span of time. The addition of operative photographs that describe the technique of endosuturing during difficult laparoscopic cholecystectomy adds additional value to the book. I am sure that the surgeons will have a thorough understanding of these techniques while they see the videos that accompany the book.

While the beginners of laparoscopic surgery will find it extremely useful as an introduction to endosuturing, surgeons who practice advanced laparoscopic surgery can also refresh their knowledge through this manual. I congratulate the authors Dr Parveen Bhatia, Dr Suviraj J John and Dr JP Singh Deed for their exhaustive work in bringing out this commendable book. I am sure that this book will definitely act as a valuable practical guide for all practicing laparoscopic surgeons.

Dr C Palanivelu

MS, MCh (GE), MNAMS, FRCS (Ed), FACS
Head of the Department of Surgical
Gastroenterology and Advanced Laparoscopic
Surgery,
Director, Gem Hospital India Ltd,
Coimbatore, Tamilnadu, India

Foreword

It gives me immense pleasure to write a Foreword for the book Step by Step Art of Endosuturing.

I have always maintained that Indian surgeons are extremely dexterous, talented and resourceful. In spite of organizational and financial constraints, centers of excellence have sprung up around the country especially in minimal access surgery. Today, India is on the Endosurgery world map due to the untiring efforts of these enterprising surgeons, who are constantly striving to expand frontiers of minimal access surgery.

The book Step by Step Art of Endosuturing is lucid and well written. It is bound to be a welcome addition in the armamentarium of surgeons practicing laparoscopy. Many surgeons have now progressed beyond basic laparoscopy and are rendering advanced laparoscopic surgical procedures. Laparoscopic suturing and tissue approximation is an area which perhaps has not received the attention it deserves.

Dr. Parveen Bhatia has been at the forefront of this surgical revolution ever since its inception more than a decade ago. I have always been impressed with this motivation, sound judgement and professional excellence. Global Hospital and Endosurgery Institute has been a landmark in the city of Delhi since its inception for exceptional services being rendered in the field of minimal access surgery. Dr Parveen Bhatia, Dr Suviraj J John and Dr JP Singh Deed have stressed on issues that are pertinent to the practicing surgeon, which makes it a ready reference manual.

With best wishes and regards.

Padamshree Dr Pradeep K Chowbey
Chairman
Department of Minimal Access Surgery
Sir Ganga Ram Hospital
New Delhi

Preface

The exponential growth of laparoscopic surgery was engendered by success of laparoscopic cholecystectomy. Despite the popularity of laparoscopic surgery, the lack of fluency in suturing and knot tying kept a wider range of laparoscopic operations at bay for many. To go beyond laparoscopic cholecystectomy and perform advanced procedures, one needs to learn techniques of securing knots, placing sutures and approximating tissues laparoscopically. Admittedly, laparoscopic suturing is difficult and complex task, but it behooves us to provide our patients with a universally adaptable technique, which utilizes readily available materials at no extra cost, and makes the procedures not only minimally invasive but also maximally effective. However it requires substantial practice for mastery.

The text will be beneficial to minimally invasive surgeons and surgeons-in-training by providing step-by-step techniques employed successfully by experts in the field. The chapters are brief and precise. Important tips and suggestions are highlighted for quick review. Few techniques detailed in the book are also available in the CD provided along with the book and are marked by ▶ . This book condenses our experience in laparoscopic suturing techniques, and it is illustrated with a selection of some 175 figures. This manual will be best utilized if it is available in the operating room, operating lounge and in the residents library.

We are grateful to our families for providing us inspiration and support. We have been benefited from the guidance of our colleagues and residents from our respective hospitals.We are very fortunate to have such outstanding support from Jaypee Brothers Medical Publishers (P) Ltd., which allows the attention to details necessary for such project.

We hope reading of these pages will enthrall the reader as much as writing them has excited us. We hope the contents will whet everyone's appetite for laparoscopic suturing techniques and encourage further education and training in this domain.

Parveen Bhatia
Suviraj J John
JP Singh Deed

Contents

1. Introduction 1

2. History 5

3. Basic Concepts 9

4. Instrumentation 25

5. Basic Technique 41

6. Intracorporeal Suturing Techniques 69

7. Intracorporeal Knot Tying 79

8. Extracorporeal Knot Tying 109

9. Common Errors and Remedies 141

10. Useful Accessories 155

11. The Future...is Here! 165

    Index 169

CD CONTENTS

1. Needle introduction inside abdomen
   (Chapter 5; p45-51)
2. Needle adjustment
   a. Needle erection (Chapter 5; p59-61)
   b. Adjustment by maneuvering suture
      (Chapter 5; p58-59)
   c. Adjustment by tip of needle
      (Chapter 5: p55-57)
3. Knotting technique
   a. Intracorporeal knotting
      I. Intracorporeal Surgeon's knot (*Live surgery*)
         Chapter 7; p88-101)
      II. Intracorporeal square knot
         (Chapter 7; p81, 82)
      III. Square slip knot (Chapter 7; p103-107)
   b. Extracorporeal knotting
      I. Roeder knot (Chapter 8; p114-123)
      II. Melzer knot (Chapter 8; p123-131)
4. Common errors and remedies
   a. Short suture length (management by 'Half
      moon effect') (Chapter 9; p146-149)
   b. Loosening of first half knot (management)
      (Chapter 9; p142-145)

Chapter 1

Introduction

It is new no matter how long we have known it. Its values crowd each other, its symbols are inexhaustible.
—*Suzan Langer*

During the early stages of a surgeon's education, the techniques of tying knots, suturing and anastomosing tissue occupy a great deal of time and effort. Indeed, progress from assistant to surgeon is predicated upon one's ability to smoothly and reliably perform these tasks.

Minimal Access Surgery could not have come in at a better time! Embraced by the public and promoted by technological advances, it has rejuvenated surgery. The excitement engendered by minimal access surgical techniques continues unabated and the speed at which operations have been performed is phenomenal.

Yet, it remains as another classic example of a 'Half-Way Technology' for a number of reasons. There is a significant learning curve associated with the various techniques of minimal access surgery (some more than the others), credentialing is not widespread, technology is still emergent or limited in many areas of minimal access surgery and last but not the least cost factors limit its widespread use.

Despite the popularity of laparoscopy in general surgery for over a decade, the lack of fluency in suturing and knot tying has kept a wider range of laparoscopic operations at bay for many. The initial enthusiasm for minimally invasive surgery was engendered by the development of laparoscopic cholecystectomy, an operation that could be performed without a single intracorporeal tie or suture. If one wishes to tackle anything other than cholecystectomy, then it is imperative that the methods of securing knots, placing sutures, and approximating tissue be learned. Indeed, it is also true that such skills may be germane to gallbladder surgery—how else might one seal a rent in the gallbladder or close a dilated cystic duct.

The clinical progress of this field is very dependent on the surgeon learning correctly the critical skills and techniques upon which the success of laparoscopic intervention hinges. Laparoscopic tissue approximation is one such critical skill that every minimal access surgeon must not only know but master! Intracorporeal suturing has, for most surgeons, remained an exotic and intimidating difficult technique. The objective of this manual is to help you simply do it flawlessly!

There are many differences between laparoscopic and open suturing. The appreciation of these differences allows surgeons to learn to adapt to the laparoscopic operating environment. The first difference is the lack of depth perception in laparoscopy, as the procedure is viewed on a two-dimensional video screen. Secondly, there is a lack of direct manual contact with the tissue. The remote technique of handling needle and thread with two instruments is considerably hampered by the length and rigidity of the instruments. It is difficult to achieve the correct needle position in the jaws of the needle holder or to drive it through the tissue in any desired direction, and it is challenging to maintain adequate suture tension. Restricted instrument mobility in laparoscopic surgery is another obstacle; for example, when passing a needle through tissue, the surgeon is confined by the cannula placement to a single arc of rotation perpendicular to the axis of the instrument. Finally, the laparoscopic view is limited to a portion of the body cavity and it is critical that instrument and needle always be followed to prevent iatrogenic injury.

The best method of tissue approximation is determined by the type of procedure being performed and the technical skills of the surgeon. These methods include intracorporeal suturing, extracorporeal knotting, endoscopic staplers, endoscopic clips, automatic suturing devices, fibrin glue, and the biofragmentable anastomosis ring.

Seek simplicity and distrust it.
—*Whitehead*

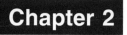

Chapter 2

History

What is now proved was once only imagined.

—*Blake*

Suturing dominated traditional open surgery for centuries. Laparoscopic suturing techniques were introduced and utilized by Semm in Gynecology in the mid-1970s.

Limitations with reference to needle, needle holder technology, slow internal knotting and difficulty in acquisition of the right level of expertise with these techniques contributed to the slow dissemination and widespread progress of laparoscopic tissue approximation.

The first significant step in the evolution of laparoscopic instruments was mating of the microsurgical handle to the laparoscopic instrument, permitting freer movement and full rotatability. Also important was the introduction of two-handed suturing techniques and the design of instruments as a matched pair (Szabo-Berci needle holders, Karl Storz Endoscopy America, Culver City, CA), with each performing its specific role of needle driving or assisting grasper. The first prototypical modification was made by bending the handle of an otolaryngology alligator grasper straight and welding a round handle in place of the ring handles.

With later development of efficient techniques of laparoscopic hand suturing, laparoscopic tissue approximation was evaluated initially in bilioenteric anastomosis and later with gastrojejunostomy and colonic resection.

In 1990, the introduction of the first endoscopic (30 mm) gastrointestinal anastomosis (GIA) stapler provided operative laparoscopists with the same efficient, safe, sutureless delivery system that we have now successfully used at laparotomy for over two decades.

Sewing devices such as the endostitch (US Surgical Corporation) has been available since 1994.

The progress in the application of these techniques in the broader context of everyday surgery remains emergent.

Chapter 3

Basic Concepts

- **UTILITY OF LAPAROSCOPIC SUTURING**
- **THE CHALLENGE**
- **PREREQUISITE FOR LAPAROSCOPIC SUTURING**
    - **Perfect Health**
    - **Visual Perception—Hand-eye Co-ordination**
    - **Motor Skill**
    - **Video Magnification and Camera Factors**
    - **Increasing Efficiency**
    - **Tissue Handling**
- **TRAINING**

A clash of doctrines is not a disaster—
it is an opportunity.

—*Whitehead*

UTILITY OF LAPAROSCOPIC SUTURING

Laparoscopic suturing and knot-tying techniques may be applied to virtually every laparoscopic operation. The surgeon may wish to use these techniques initially under non-urgent conditions by replacing other tissue approximation modalities. For instance, during a laparoscopic cholecystectomy, the surgeon can ligate the cystic duct and artery or close a gallbladder perforation using manual suturing or knot-tying techniques rather than resorting to an automatic clip applier or a pre-formed slip knot. During laparoscopic appendectomy, rather than using one of the disposable linear staplers (Endo-GIA, US Surgical) to ligate and divide the appendiceal mesentery and base of the appendix, one might use pre-formed slip knots or ligate the mesentery in continuity using interrupted sutures and external square knots set with a pushrod. As the surgeon advances to other laparoscopic operations, many other applications of these basic surgical skills become apparent. For repair of hiatal hernia, either running or interrupted sutures may be used for the fundoplication. When confronted with unsuspected common bile duct stones that cannot be removed via the cystic duct, a choledochotomy can be performed and then closed using fine sutures tied intracorporeally. When the technique of bowel resection is perfected, it will be imperative for surgeons to utilize laparoscopic suturing skills.

We acknowledge that many instrument manufactures are developing laparoscopic staplers to facilitate bowel anastomoses. However, laparoscopic suturing and knot-tying skills will be necessary to close defects in a staple line, to place purse-string sutures for end-to-end stapling, to close mesenteric defects, or to ligate large blood vessels with something more satisfactory than a clip. As with open surgery, the surgeon must learn and practice these basic surgical skills until they become second nature and can be employed whenever needed.

Laparoscopic suturing techniques can be used for tying cystic duct and artery, appendiceal mesentry and appendix, repair of hiatal hernia, fundoplication and choledochotomy closure etc.

THE CHALLENGE

Today, a wide variety of tissue approximation techniques are available laparoscopically. The initial use of traditional suturing in laparoscopic procedures was difficult and discouraging, too, resulting in a need for alternate methods of approximation. However, despite its technical challenges, intracorporeal laparoscopic suturing continues to be the preferred technique of laparoscopic tissue approximation.

The greatest obstacle in laparoscopic suturing is the lack of skill, but this can be overcome by proper technique, training and instrumentation. It needs time, dexterity and constant practice. There are many differences between open and laparoscopic suturing. The appreciation of these differences allows surgeons to learn to adapt to the laparoscopic operating environment.

1. Lack of direct manual contact with tissue.
2. Lack of depth perception.
3. Restricted instrument mobility.
4. Limitation of laparoscopic view to a portion of the body cavity.

Given the present state of technology, there are a number of factors that restrict one's ability to tie knots and place sutures laparoscopically, and an appreciation of these problems allows one to modify or adapt the techniques to optimize proficiency and speed. The first technical difference between laparoscopic and open surgery is that, in laparoscopy—there is a lack of direct manual contact with the tissue. One's sense of 'feel' is restricted to that which is transmitted via a 30-cm-long instrument. The second difference is that the surgeon is not viewing the laparoscopic field with direct binocular vision. Rather, the image is transmitted to a two-dimensional video screen, and the laparoscope magnifies the image to as much as 18 times its normal size. The magnification accentuates a person's natural tremor, and the two-dimensional view eliminates true depth perception. One must find the distance between the end of the telescope and tissue at which there is apparent depth perception, especially when using visual clues provided by instruments manipulated in the field. When operating from a video screen, it is imperative not to look at one's hands during the actual procedure, a concept that is difficult for many surgeons to internalize. With practice, a certain measure of video-eye-hand coordination is cultivated. These are learned skills, rather than innate tendencies, that improve over time.

Lack of sense of 'feel' and depth perception, makes task of laparoscopic suturing more difficult.

Another fundamental difference between laparoscopic and open surgery is that there is restricted instrument mobility with the former. The sites for the laparoscopic sheaths are mobile only to the limited degree of elasticity of the abdominal wall itself. When passing a needle through tissue, the surgeon is confined by the trocar placement to a single arc of rotation perpendicular to the axis of the instrument. Certainly, additional trocars may be inserted when necessary, but the surgeon should plan so as to place the cannulae in optimal positions. The instrument ports should not be too close to one another, to the optic, or to the operating field, nor should they parlay one another. The accessory instrument cannulae should be spaced with an intertrocar distance of at least 5 cm to avoid "sword fighting." The operating ports must be positioned to ensure that the working tips of the instruments meet in the operative field at oblique angles to one another. The distance between the site of cannula entry and the operative field should equal about half the length of the instruments used for tissue approximation: Because most instruments are 30 cm in length, this would equal 15 cm from entry site to the operative field. If a third cannula is necessary, it should be sited primarily with a view to optimal retraction of the surrounding tissue.

Positioning of video screen, port placement, angle between instruments and depth of insertion of instruments makes critical difference as there is restricted space for working.

The tip of the instrument with which one is working must be in front of the laparoscope, and the surgeon's eyes should be directed in line with the video screen. The instruments should enter the field of view tangentially rather than in a coaxial orientation, or the instruments themselves will obscure the operative field. If at all possible, the instruments should advance out of the sheaths toward the video screen and away from the laparoscope; attempts at operating with the instruments advancing toward the laparoscope and away from the video screen lead to great frustration as one attempts to operate under "mirror vision."

When performing laparoscopic cholecystectomy, it is extremely easy to become a "one-handed" surgeon. Instruments placed through a single operating port may be manipulated with the dominant hand while stabilizing the laparoscopic sheath with the nondominant hand. For suturing and knot tying, two-handed manipulation is necessary, and this often requires an assistant to stabilize the laparoscopic cannulae or, alternatively, to use one of the new laparoscopic ports with fixation devices such as screw threads or inflatable sub-peritoneal balloons.

The skill level required for various surgical modalities has been detailed below (Fig. 3.1):
- Conventional surgery - 1.5 points on a scale of 10.
- Micro-surgery   - 4   points on a scale of 10.

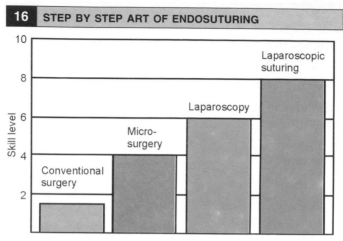

Fig. 3.1: A relative comparison of skill required for various surgical modalities

- Laparoscopy   - 6 points on a scale of 10.
- Laparoscopic suturing - 8 points on a scale of 10.

The results suggest that the use of videoendoscopic techniques requires a greater intensity of physical effort than open surgery techniques.

PREREQUISITE FOR LAPAROSCOPIC SUTURING

Perfect Health

The slowed choreography of intracorporeal suturing requires considerable patience and fresh energy. It is recommended:

- Be in top physical and mental condition. Energy limits can be increased by-
  - Sportsman-like lifestyle

- Conditioning
- Discipline
- That one abstains from caffeine and other stimulants.
- It is also vital to avoid mental and physical distractions in the operating room and other factors that dilute concentration, e.g. mobile phone.

LESSON
1. Get in shape.
2. Avoid stimulants and distractions.

Visual Perception Hand-eye Co-ordination

- Good visual health, correction to 20/20 vision and rested eyes are components of the ideal physical and mental conditioning required in laparoscopic suturing. It has been observed during microsurgical training that slight visual flaws that do not disturb surgeons during open surgery become problematic when looking at a magnified surgical field. A visit to the ophthalmologist is recommended before taking a laparoscopic course or proceeding to operate with the aid of magnification.
- Visual magnification enhances visual perception resulting in a more precise, and convenient repair. However, this enhanced visual perception results in a hand-eye co-ordination imbalance that must be compensated by:

- Slowing movements until proper control is re-established.
- Changing magnification according to the activity. Important decisions need greater magnification and focus.

The importance of proper training is obvious because building up a good visual memory and concurrent reasoning allows the surgeon to read poor quality visual clues correctly.

Proficiency in specific aspects of visual perception is directly associated with performance speed on dexterity drills, shown in previous studies to be fundamental in the development of intracorporeal suturing skill.[1]

LESSON
1. Rest eyes; get them checked if laparoscopic surgery is disturbed.
2. Slow movements until proper control is gained.
3. Get properly trained from the beginning.

Motor Skill

Motor skill determines the performance of a successful surgical procedure. The balance and coordination of perception, decision making and motor skill orchestrate the ideal procedure. Because laparoscopic surgery requires adjustment to a magnified field, the motor skills that we have developed over a life time in everyday practice are distorted. Magnification and the use of foot-long instrumentation create an imbalance. This is compensated by a special approach that is commonly referred to as principles of microsurgery. Familiarity with open microsurgery eases the transition from open traditional surgery to laparoscopic surgery.

LESSON
Adhere to the principles of microsurgery.

Video Magnification and Camera Factors

A well tuned high-quality set-up will provide a video picture that is adequate for most suturing procedures. The most frequently used magnification is 3x to 4x (range 1x to 15x). This relatively low level of magnification is equivalent to the low range of the surgical microscope and the working range of loupes. In microsurgery, this requires only moderate adaptation in surgical technique. In laparoscopic surgery, the length of the instrumentation multiplies the degree of difficulty and proportionately greater adaptation is needed.

- Adjusting the image for sharpness and clarity is vital. Sustained concentration on the video screen can cause eye strain.

- The camera assistant is instrumental in providing the best visual image because holding and guiding the camera is one of the most difficult roles performed by the operating team. The task of keeping the lens clean and making sure the image remains focused is difficult to maintain for more than 30 minutes, particularly when the procedure is not going smoothly. It is useful to rotate jobs of camera holding from time to time. The other alternative is to utilize a camera holder-First Assistant (Leonard Medical, Huntingdon Valley, Pa) or the Lapo Tract M.I.S. Support system (Omni-Tract Surgical, St. Paul, MN).

- The optimal ergonomic conditions include an endoscope-to-target distance of 75-150 mm. The direction of view of the endoscope has no significant effect on intracorporeal knotting if the optical axis subtended the same angle with the task surface.[2]

- A range of 60-90 degrees manipulation angles with equal azimuth angles is recommended. As the manipulation angle increases, the elevation angle has to increase accordingly.[3]

LESSON
Adjust for excellent resolution and position.

Increasing Efficiency

Reducing speed to counter hand-eye coordination imbalance can lengthen operating time, which is counter-productive, considering anaesthesia time and operating costs. Combining the following important principles can increase efficiency:

- Economy of motion principle
- Ergonomics
- Choreography-of-movements technique
- Precision control in movement of instrument tip

For example, knotting movements have been studied and choreographed into the least number of necessary movements that flow into one another smoothly. The ultimate goal for the surgeon is to develop a flawless technique.

The better task performance by expert surgeons is associated with controlled rapid manipulations and a wider range of movement at the shoulder joint of the dominant upper limb.[4]

LESSON

Practice the above-mentioned principles religiously.

Tissue Handling

This is a major concern in minimal access surgery and

especially in intra-corporeal suturing. The need for delicate tissue handling cannot be overstressed.

- Provide safe retraction.
- Avoid collateral trauma.
- Use instruments for their intended function only. Avoid interchange.
- Tissues need to be handled as gently as possible, especially when being positioned for needle passage.
- Counter pressure should be provided immediately adjacent to the point of needle entrance or exit by the jaws of the assisting grasper.
- Minor adjustments and initial testing of tissue can be made with the tip of a needle firmly held in the grip of the needle driver.
- A good set-up facilitates the entire procedure. Tissue edges needing to be approximated if brought in close proximity makes suturing a straight-forward process.
- Extra set of "Hands" may be needed.

TRAINING

For the new surgeons, suturing and knot tying skills will be incorporated into residency programs. For practicing surgeons, a dedicated course of study will be the first step and should be followed by regular practice.

Key factors to success are:
- Motivation
- Willpower
- Discipline

To develop a competent confident technique, one must approach training to perform intracorporeal suturing in a manner similar to training for an athletic competition.

After didactic presentations, much can be accomplished with inanimate models. Initially, the surgeon should become familiar with the instruments and sutures (hardware so to speak). Placing pre-tied Roeder loops on foam models and then practicing extra-corporeal Roeder knot is a good first step.

Animal models are suitable for practicing ties on vessels, such as those that supply the porcine spleen or for closing induced gastric perforations. One can finely hone the techniques to fashion sutured or stapled anastomosis in animals, although some of the newer inanimate models are also well suited for this training.

Currently, virtual reality technique (MIST-VR) is being utilised for training and has been found to superior in few studies.[5,6]

Thinking is more interesting than knowing, but less interesting than looking.

—Goethe

REFERENCES

1. Risucci D, Geiss A, Gellman L et al. Experience and visual perception in resident acquisition of laparoscopic skills. Curr Surg. 2000 Jul 1; 57(4): 368-372.
2. Hanna GB, Shimi S, Cuschieri A. Influence of direction of view, target-to-endoscope distance and manipulation angle on endoscopic knot tying. Br J Surg. 1997 Oct; 84(10): 1460-4.
3. Hanna GB, Shimi S, Cuschieri A. Optimal port locations for endoscopic intracorporeal knotting. Surg Endosc. 1997 Apr; 11(4): 397-401.
4. Emam TA, Hanna GB, Kimber C et al. Differences between experts and trainees in the motion pattern of the dominant upper limb during intracorporeal endoscopic knotting. Dig Surg. 2000; 17(2): 120-3; discussion 124-5.
5. Grantcharov TP, Kristiansen VB, Bendix J, et al. Randomized clinical trial of virtual reality simulation for laparoscopic skills training. Br J Surg 2004 Feb;91(2):146-50.
6. Seymour NE, Gallagher AG, Roman SA, et al. Virtual reality training improves operating room performance: Results of a randomized, double-blinded study. Ann Surg 2002 Oct; 236(4):458-63; discussion 463-4.

Instrumentation

- **TROCARS**
- **NEEDLE AND SUTURE**
  - **Needle Characteristics**
  - **Suture Characteristics**
- **ENDOLOOPS**
- **HAND INSTRUMENTS**
  - **Needle Holder**
  - **First Generation (Semm) Needle Holders—5 mm and 3 mm**
  - **Second Generation Needle Holders (Ethicon, Cook and Wolfe)**
  - **Throw Pushers**
  - **Grasping Forceps**

Mechanical excellence is the only vehicle of genius.
—*Blake*

Suturing is one of the key problems of endoscopic surgery. The remote technique of handling needle and thread with two instruments is considerably hampered by the length and rigidity of the instruments. It is difficult to achieve the correct needle position in the jaws or to drive it through the tissue in any desired direction.

This chapter explains the principles involved in the design, configuration and construction of these essential implements of surgical operative practice. In addition to the correct technique, specific suturing tasks require special needles and suture materials for optimum results. A working knowledge of the physical principles behind the various needle configurations and an awareness of the mechanical, biological and surgical characteristics of the available range of suture materials, therefore, underlies correct selective usage.

Special considerations apply to suturing techniques in endoscopic surgery which impose restrictions on the ergonomic maneuverability and visual perspective display problems not encountered in conventional open surgery. These materially influence the choice of needle and suture materials used, as undoubtedly the selection of the correct combination for the intended surgical task facilitates the conduct of the endoscopic procedure in addition to optimizing the end result.

TROCARS

- Ideally trocars should be just a little longer than the thickness of the abdominal wall.
- Long trocar interferes with instrument mobility and function.
- Preferred diameter is 10-11mm, permitting passage of curved needles and a variety of instruments.
- Temporary fixation to the abdominal wall is desirable.
- A frequent problem are reducer caps, often requiring two hands to replace while changing instruments or passing needle through.

NEEDLE AND SUTURE

- Proper selection of suture is critical. Each surgical procedure requires specific needle configurations and needle and thread combinations.

Needle Characteristics

- Handling characteristics—Ideal needle should have a bicurve geometry. Different sites require different needle sizes.
- The tip—The tapered needle with a small cutting tip is ideal.

- Diameter and profile of the needle—The grip should be a well-matched, refined grip. Thicker tissue layers require sturdier needles; more delicate tissues require smaller thinner needles.

The *straight needle* (Fig. 4.1) was earlier handled by the Semm needle holder. Straight round bodied needle has limited use with friable tissue and can easily tear tissue at its point of entry.

The *Ski-shaped needle* (Fig. 4.2) are rounded near the slightly curved tip and triangular along the straight shaft (Ethicon, USSC). The needle is gripped along the triangular shaft and avoids the problem of swivel. Improved 'Ski' needles with flattened cross-section (Dundee) (Fig. 4.4) along the shaft can be easily erected by simply grasping them. The flat cross-section has another advantage: the locking is improved, which increases the fixation of jaws.

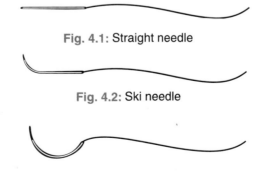

Fig. 4.1: Straight needle

Fig. 4.2: Ski needle

Fig. 4.3: Curved needle

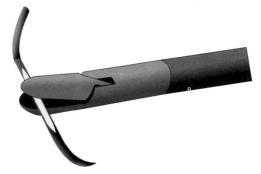

Fig. 4.4: 'Ski' needles with flattened cross-section (Dundee)

The standard *curved needles* (Fig. 4.3) are good alternative to the Ski needles, however, the needle can swivel during suturing.

Suture Characteristics

- Should have a favorable tissue response.
- Good handling/memory characteristics—2-0, 3-0 silk is easiest to handle and tie a secure knot. Roeder knot has best results with chromic catgut but is not suitable for PDS or polypropylene.
- Coloring—A pitch black or fluorescent white (PTFE or Gore-tex) color are unanimous favorites.
- For intracorporeal interrupted or running sutures and specifically for intracorporeal knotting, a polyfilament suture should be used.
- Extracorporeal slipknots tied with silk and polyamide have been found to be less secure than the

equivalent knots tide with Dacron, lactomer, and polydioxanone.
- Prelooped intracorporeal knot is available which renders intracorporeal knotting an easy and rapid task to achieve.[1]

ENDOLOOPS

Pre-formed slip knots are also available commercially and packaged as the Endoloop (Ethicon, Inc., New Brunswick, NJ) or the Surgitie (US Surgical, Inc., Norwalk, CT). The suture is packaged with the long tail of the loop threaded through a plastic pushrod, the end of which is snapped off to release the tail of the suture. This slip knot is useful for ligating structures that have already been divided or for closing holes in structures in which the two opposing edges of the defect can be grasped and drawn together:
- The endoloop is drawn backward into a 5 to 3 mm reducer.
- After the endoloop is introduced into the abdominal cavity, a grasper is passed through it and holds the tubular structure until the endoloop knot is pushed into position.
- The pushrod is then broken and inserted to tighten the loop down around the base of the structure while the tissue itself is picked up and placed on tension inside the loop.

UTILITY

This technique works well for closing perforations of the gallbladder wall, for ligating the base of the appendix, for closure of a wide cystic duct, and for ligating bleeding vessels on the free margin of the omentum.

Similarly, a ligature can also be applied in continuity with a commercially available suture and plastic pusher.

- The thread is passed into the body cavity through a 3 to 5 mm reducer.
- Then maneuvered around the structure and back out through the reducer.
- A knot is effected externally and pushed into position with the plastic pushing device.
- A thread with a pre-applied needle can also be used.
- The needle is passed through the tissue and brought out through the reducer.
- The knot is fashioned externally and pushed back inside.

HAND INSTRUMENTS

Needle Holder

The primary role of the needle holder/driver is handling the needle, although suturing and tissue grasping are also part of its functions.

- A slight spooning curvature is the preferred shape of the tip.
- For grasping tissue and looping suture, the tip must be able to reach in almost any direction. This is best accomplished with an aggressively curved or angled tip, for example a flamingo beak-shaped tip.
- Jaw should be finely engineered so that it grasps fine sutures without slipping,
- Rounded edges to avoid accidental cutting of the suture, as traction is applied.
- The dominant needle holder should have a lock that the surgeon can activate or inactivate at will.
- It should be strong and preferably have one moving jaw (to reduce suture snagging).
- The lock on the non-dominant needle holder should preferably be inactivated.
- The best quality of laparoscopic bowel suturing, in terms of the accuracy of suture placement and the integrity of the suture line closure, can be obtained with a 40 degrees handle-to-shaft angle.[2]

First Generation (Semm) Needle Holders— 5 mm and 3 mm

The standard Semm needle holders (Figs 4.5 and 4.6) have handles that are at right angle to the shaft, and working jaws of the tip have a serrated surface. It provides secure manipulation of a straight round bodied needle. These holders allow curved needles to swivel and, because of the orientation of the handle, the extent of the wrist motion during suturing is exaggerated.

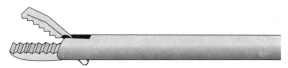

Fig. 4.5: Semm needle holder (5 mm)

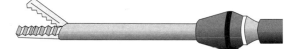

Fig. 4.6: Semm needle holder (3 mm)

Advantages

1. Needle is easily oriented.
2. Grasped without the risk of needle rotation as might be the case with a curved needle.
3. Secure grip.

Disadvantages

1. Oblique grasping is not possible.
2. In areas where space is confined, straight needle is difficult to manipulate.
3. Curved needles swivel and loose orientation.
4. Wrist movements are exaggerated due to handle design.

Second Generation Needle Holders (Ethicon, Cook and Wolfe)

Newer needle holders have different grasping mechanism with improved jaw design and serrations (diamond shaped). The handles are inline with the shaft or the handles that can be opened from any rotational angle (similar to Castro-Viejo needle holders). These allow for much more secure grasping of standard flattened needle shafts and have paved the way for the use of standard curved needles. Introduction of the curved needle requires the diameter of the larger 11 mm port. To improve the delicate handling of both the grip and the locking mechanism classical and novel design features have been introduced.

The most advanced mechanism created by **Wolf** (Fig. 4.7) involves telescopic locking which functions like a ball point pen; one pressing locks and the next releases the grip. Unfortunately, the mechanism cannot be disassembled, which hinders complete and easy cleaning.

The **Cook** curved needle holder (Fig. 4.8) has an altogether different jaw design which automatically sets the curved needle in upright position and certainly has the advantage of grasping the needle securely but suffers from being a bit awkward to regrasp the needle. However, only one needle position is possible with a particular type of Cook needle holder and there is difficulty of internal handling of suture.

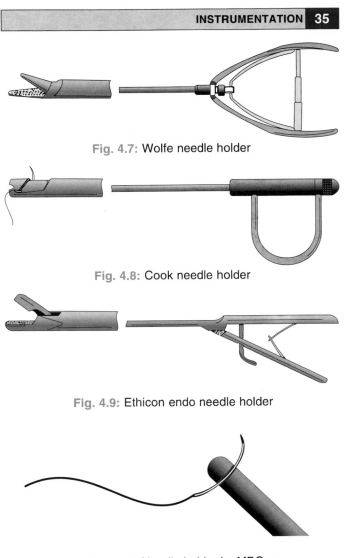

Fig. 4.7: Wolfe needle holder

Fig. 4.8: Cook needle holder

Fig. 4.9: Ethicon endo needle holder

Fig. 4.10: Needle holder by MBG

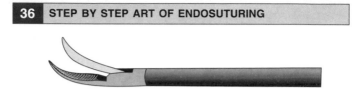

Fig. 4.11: Szabo and Berci needle holder
(Flamingo shaped)

The needle holder by MBG (Gembloux, Belgium, Fig. 4.10) probably has the firmest gripping of the holders available. Its principle is quite simple; it consists of a tube and a pushrod and two tungsten metal rings which are simple pressed against each other. There are two major disadvantages to design; it is difficult to tie a knot, because the tip is too long and the opening depth of jaws is reduced due to the central rod.

Z. Szabo and G. Berci have designed two instruments, the parrot and the flamingo forceps (Fig. 4.11), which permit excellent execution of internal suturing and knotting. Although, the handling is not optimal, the congruently shaped jaws of the instruments facilitate grasping and positioning of needle and thread. The handle is designed like a Castro-Viejo needle holder and can be opened from any rotational position. The axial shape enables rotation of the instrument 360 degrees which allows the precise maneuvering necessary for laparoscopic suturing.

NEEDLE HOLDER/DRIVER

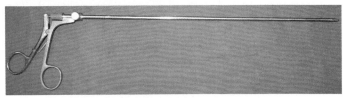

Fig. 4.12: Needle holder (Pistol type handles)

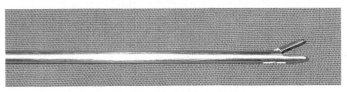

Fig. 4.13: Needle holder: Jaws open

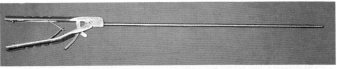

Fig. 4.14: Self-righting needle holder (Coaxial handle design)

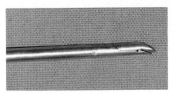

Fig. 4.15: Self-righting needle holder (Observe the notch)

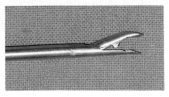

Fig. 4.16: Self-righting needle holder: Jaws open

A disposable suture applier called **Lapromed** consists of a needle, suture, pre-tied knot and applicator. The needle with the thread is stored in the tip of the device. After introduction, the needle can be grasped. It is attached to a 15 cm (6 inches) long thread. The knot is pretied and two loops are exposed at the tip of the shaft. To make these slip knots the needle is simply led through those two loops and the knot can then be fastened from outside by means of a retraining band.

Latest improvements include the addition of the 'needle self-righting property' to the jaws of the needle holder (Figs 4.14 to 4.16). They allow the needle to erect in upright position automatically and at right angles to the jaws for convenient suturing.

Two needle holders may be used for laparoscopic suturing or one may use a grasper in non-dominant hand.

There are many patterns of needle holders available. Besides the variety mentioned above, the handle design may be pistol type (Figs 4.12 and 4.13) or coaxial (Fig. 4.14). The surgeon should try those that are available and find which suits his or her preferences.

Throw Pushers

During extracorporeal suturing the knot (or the throw) must be pushed into the abdominal cavity and set tight with the help of knot pusher.

The surgeon should have both 5 and 3 mm throw pushers to lay external throws. Plastic (Fig. 4.17) and metal pushers (Fig. 4.18) are commercially available that are designed to push external ties of 0 and 2-0 suture material inside the body cavity. A variety of knot pushers are available, including those with a slit circle in the end or forceps with notched tips that can be used to push down the knot.

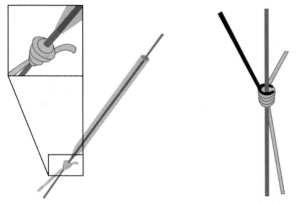

Fig. 4.17: Plastic knot pusher   Fig. 4.18: Metal knot pusher

Most of the reusable knot pushers have grooves, small terminal slits or forks and all of them tend to lose the thread when the knot is pushed down. All disposable pushers consist of a simple plastic tube. Although, it is impossible to lose the thread, reinserting a thread through the long rod is difficult.

Grasping Forceps

The grasping forceps mainly acts as an assisting instrument.

It:

- Handles tissues and sutures.
- Provides counter pressure.
- Performs a minimal role in needle driving.
- In special cases, it can also hold and drive the needle (Ambidextrous approach).

Certain specifications are desirable in the tissue grasper—

- Tip should be curved ideally, which allows tissue and needle grasping.
- Jaw hinge design may be single or twin action.
- Engineering of jaw hinge should be such to avoid snaring of suture.

Trainer

A trainer with a self-stabilizing camera is essential for practice. Virtual reality trainers (MIST-VR) make training quicker and convenient.

REFERENCES

1. Nouira Y, Horchani A. The pre-looped intracorporeal knot: a new technique for knot tying in laparoscopic surgery. J Urol 2001 Jul; 166(1): 195-7.
2. Ahmed S, Hanna GB, Cuschieri A. Optimal angle between instrument shaft and handle for laparoscopic bowel suturing. Arch Surg 2004 Jan; 139(1): 89-92.

Chapter 5

Basic Technique

- **SET UP**
  - **Laparoscope and Instrument Location**
  - **Principles of Port Placement**
  - **Principles of Instrumentation**
- **NEEDLE CONTROL**
  - **Introduction of Needle Inside Abdomen**
  - **Loading the Needle**
  - **Adjusting the Needle**
  - **Driving the Needle**
- **ENTRANCE AND EXIT BITES**
  - **Selection of Entrance Point**
  - **Amount of Bite**
  - **Exit Bite**

Reason can ascertain the profound difficulties of our condition, it cannot remove them.

—*Newman*

SET UP

Laparoscope and Instrument Location

- Positioning the camera through the umbilicus is sufficient for most procedures, although it can be changed to accommodate the need for special access.
- There are two models of positioning:
  1. The natural position of the surgeon:
     - The laparoscope is located between the right and left instruments (Fig. 5.1).
  2. The offset position
     - The instrument pair located to one side of the laparoscope.

     The natural position is more convenient and ergonomically better.
- Optimal laparoscopic suturing (better task quality and reduced execution time) is achieved with *vertical* suturing toward the surgeon with iso-planar monitor display of the operative field. The poorer task performance observed during *horizontal* suturing is accompanied by more muscle work and fatigue, and it is not improved by monitor display of the enterotomy in the vertical plane.[1]

Principles of Port Placement

- Ideally the needle driver should be lined up parallel to the proposed suture line. The assisting grasper should be offset at least 60 to 90 degrees (manipulation angle) (Figs 5.1 and 5.2) and set 6-7 inches apart to avoid a 'Chopstick' effect.

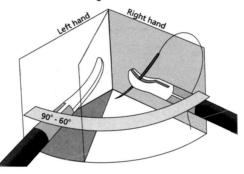

Fig. 5.1: Ideal positioning of the needle driver and the assisting grasper is a 60- to 90- degrees angle (Manipulation angle)

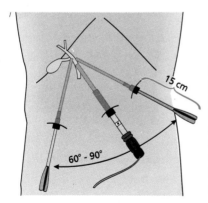

Fig. 5.2: The ideal port position for closure of a choledochotomy spreads the needle holder and assisting forceps by 60 degrees to 90 degrees with one-half of the instrument (15 cm) in the patient and one-half out

- An alternative way for correct port placement is to make an isosceles triangle between the instruments with an angle between 25 degrees to 45 degrees and an angle of < 55 degrees between the instruments and the horizontal line as the optimal geometry for intracorporeal suturing. These data should be considered when planning a reconstructive laparoscopic procedure.[2]

- Whenever possible, laparoscopic surgeons should strive to place their instruments and trocars so as to minimize extreme horizontal or vertical displacement of their hands away from a resting position of comfort.[3]

Principles of Instrumentation

- Better endoscopic task performance and more ergonomic movements of a surgeon's dominant upper limb can be achieved within a certain range of intracorporeal-extracorporeal instrument length ratio. Intracorporeal-extracorporeal instrument length ratio below 1.0 degrades task performance and is associated with a wider range of movement at the elbow and shoulder and a higher angular velocity at the shoulder. An almost equal intracorporeal to extracorporeal instrument ratio is, hence, used for most instruments (Fig. 5.2). Since standard length of instruments is 30 cm, approximate intracorporeal/extracorporeal length is 15 cm.[4]

- A distance of 75-150 mm between endoscope tip and target is optimal ergonomic condition for suturing.

- Optimum conditions for good suturing include *needle holding angle* >90 degrees and *angle of needle insertion into tissues of* 80 degrees to 100 degrees. The needle should be gripped at the junction of middle and proximal third of the shaft.[5]

NEEDLE CONTROL

Introduction of Needle Inside Abdomen

1. Using 5 mm reducer
2. Percutaneous
3. Through 5 mm port (Reich method)
4. Through 10 mm port

1. Using 5 mm Reducer ▶

- Thread the needle holder through the 5 mm reducer (Fig. 5.5).

- Hold the suture somewhere near the centre with the help of needle holder (Fig. 5.6).

- Gently backload the needle holder out of reducer while maintaining grasp on the suture. This maneouver draws the suture along with needle inside the reducer (Fig. 5.7).

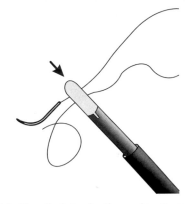

Fig. 5.3: Needle introduction using 5 mm reducer

- Continue to withdraw the needle holder till the needle and the suture are fully concealed inside the reducer (Fig. 5.8).
- Now, introduce the assembly of reducer, needle holder and suture into the 10 mm port (Fig. 5.9).
- Once fully inside the 10 mm port, gently advance the needle holder inside the abdomen, thereby exposing the suture and later the needle, under vision (Fig. 5.10 and 5.11).
- Grasp the suture with a second instrument.
- The needle and suture are ready for use.

NEEDLE INTRODUCTION USING 5 mm REDUCER

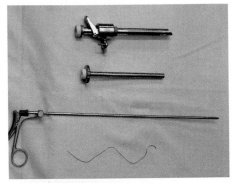

Fig. 5.4: Equipment needed for needle introduction

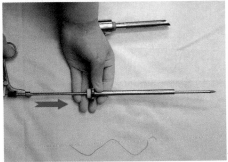

Fig. 5.5: Introduce the needle holder through the 5 mm reducer

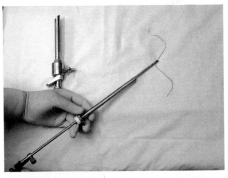

Fig. 5.6: Hold the suture in the middle with needle holder

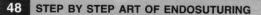

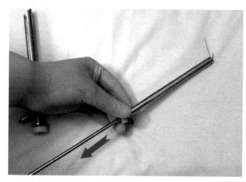

Fig. 5.7: Backload the needle holder taking the suture and needle inside the reducer

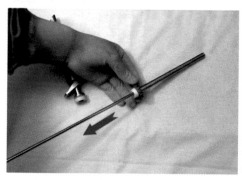

Fig. 5.8: Withdraw, till the needle is completely inside

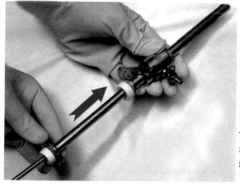

Fig. 5.9: Introduce the needle holder—5 mm reducer—suture assembly in 10 mm port

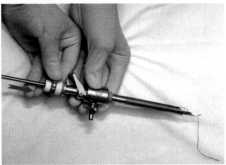

Fig. 5.10: Advance the needle holder to expose the suture (inside the abdomen)

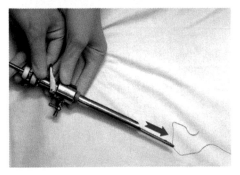

Fig. 5.11: Needle and suture in their destination (safely inside abdomen)

NEEDLE INTRODUCTION

- Hold the suture in the middle with needle holder which has already been threaded into 5 mm reducer and backload the needle holder.
- Introduce the needle holder—5 mm reducer—suture assembly in 10 mm port.
- Advance the needle holder to expose the needle inside the abdomen.

NEEDLE INTRODUCTION USING 5 mm REDUCER
(ALTERNATE TECHNIQUE)

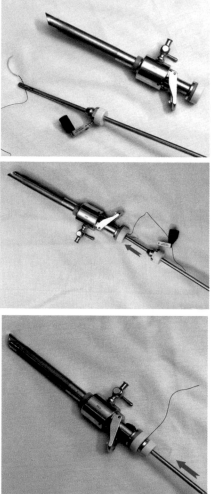

Fig. 5.12: Catch the suture near the needle with the needle holder, after introducing it in a 5 mm reducer

Fig. 5.13: Introduce the needle holder in the 10 mm port

Fig. 5.14: Advance the needle holder inside the 10 mm port

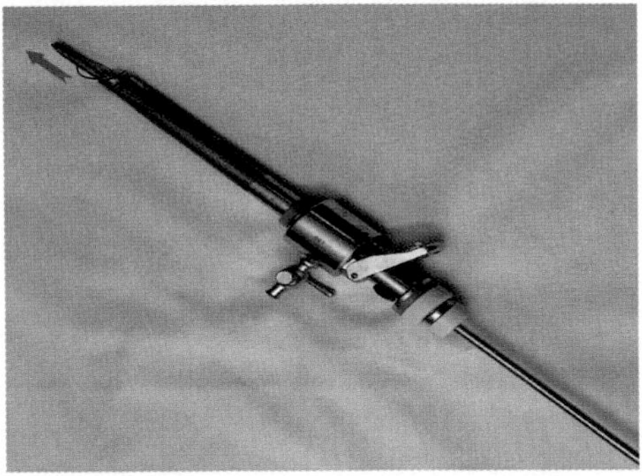

Fig. 5.15: Advance further to expose the
needle and suture

2. Percutaneous

Only applicable for straight needle and large curved
needles, especially in thin or pediatric patients.

3. Using 5 mm Port (Reich method)

- Under endovision observe the position of the tip
  of the 5 mm port and ensure that it is in a safe
  position away from the vital structures.
- Pull the 5 mm port out of the abdomen.
- Introduce the needle holder through the 5 mm port
  (outside the abdomen) and grasp the suture
  (required to be passed inside) somewhere near the
  needle.
- Introduce the needle holder percutaneously
  through the tract of the 5 mm port while
  maintaining similar direction for passing.

- Watch the entry of needle holder along with the suture via endovision.
- Once the needle holder along with the suture and the needle are completely inside the abdomen, railroad the 5 mm port over the needle holder.
- The suture is now ready for deployment.

CAUTION
- While forcing the needle along with the needle holder inside the abdomen through the 5 mm port tract, the needle may inadvertently break off from the suture. Be gentle while pushing.
- Direction of passing through abdominal wall should be same as 5 mm port, else it can get stuck in the parietal wall; injury can occur.

4. Using 10 mm Port

The position of the camera is generally at the 10 mm port. The same port can be used for introduction of the needle. This method is very useful when large needle needs to be introduced. Such needles may not possibly be concealed inside a 5 mm reducer.

- Through endovision observe the structures in the path of, and directly under the 10 mm port. Position the port direction in such a manner that no vital structure are in close proximity of the port.
- Withdraw the camera out of the 10 mm port.

- Introduce a needle holder (holding the suture from somewhere near the needle) through the 10 mm port and advance it to a distance, so that the tip of the needle holder is just exposed out of the port. While this maneouver is being done, the assistant maintains the port in the same direction and orientation.

- Release the grasp over the needle and withdraw the needle holder leaving the needle and the sutures inside.

- Introduce the camera and concentrate on the needle. Also try to look for any inadvertent injury caused by the needle.

CAUTION
- While introducing the needle/suture can get stuck in the valve of the port.
- To prevent any inadvertent injury the assistant must maintain same direction and orientation of the port throughout the maneuver.
- It is blind procedure. Do not insert the needle holder deeply inside the abdomen. Introduce it to depth just sufficient to expose the needle holder tip outside the port (intraabdominally), else injury can occur.

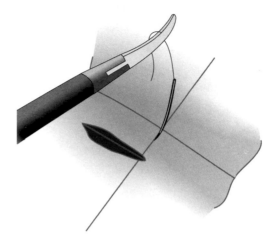

Fig. 5.16: Ideal tip alignment is gained by picking the suture up by the tail and pirouetting the needle on the tissue surface

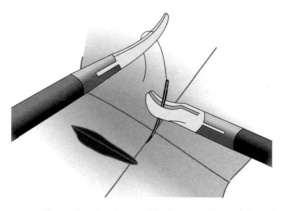

Fig. 5.17: Grasping is done with the needle holder when proper alignment is achieved

Loading the Needle

- First grasp the thread about an inch from the needle with the assisting grasper (Fig. 5.16).
- Dangle it in a fashion so that the tip of the needle touches the tissue surface.
- The needle is rotated and pivoted until it lines up in the exact direction needed (Fig. 5.17).
- It is then grasped with the needle driver.
- Gripping at the junction of middle and proximal third of the shaft of the needle is optimum for good suturing.
- Optimum conditions for good suturing include *needle holding angle* >90 degrees and *angle of needle insertion into tissues of* 80 degrees to 100 degrees.[5]
- Tip to tip method: Should the tip of needle be seen by taking the tip of the scope close to the needle so that exact direction is known.

Adjusting the Needle

Beginners will attempt to reposition the needle by handling it back and forth between assisting grasper and needle driver, hoping to adjust it in the process. This technique might seem logical; but it requires considerable skill and can turn into a frustrating "catch me if you can" situation.

- A better method is to hook the needle tip into the tissue just lightly enough to fix it, loosening the

NEEDLE ADJUSTMENT BY TIP

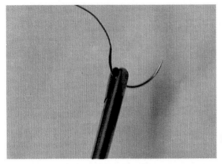

Fig. 5.18: Mal-aligned needle

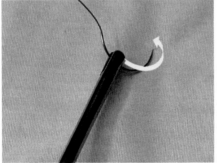

Fig. 5.19: Hook the tip of needle in solid tissue. Adjust the needle by momentarily releasing the grip and moving the needle holder till correct alignment is reached

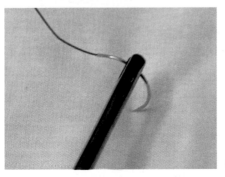

Fig. 5.20: Correct alignment achieved

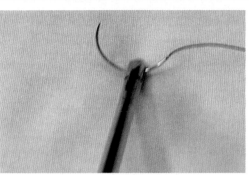

Fig. 5.21: Aligned needle ready for suturing

NEEDLE ADJUSTMENT BY TIP
- Hook the tip of needle in solid tissue viz. muscle/fascia.
- Release grip.
- Adjust orientation.
- Regrip and start suturing.

grip on the needle without actually letting it go, then pushing, pulling, or rotating the needle driver to pivot the needle into the desired position. This will need skill and concentration (Figs 5.18 to 5.21). ▶

- Another method is grasping the needle lightly and brushing it backward against tissues, this movement will sweep the point of the needle exactly opposite of the direction it is pushed.

NEEDLE ADJUSTMENT BY MANEUVERING SUTURE

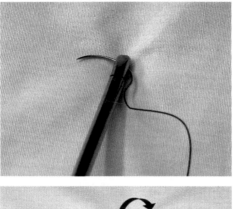

Fig. 5.22: Mal-aligned needle

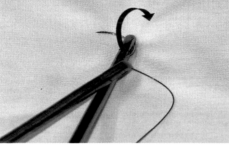

Fig. 5.23: Hold the suture near the swaged end and adjust the needle by maneuvering suture

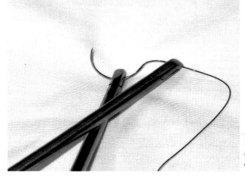

Fig. 5.24: Needle aligned by maneuvering the suture

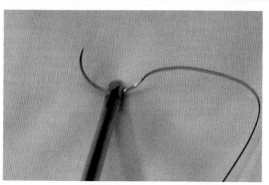

Fig. 5.25: Well aligned needle, ready for suturing

NEEDLE ADJUSTMENT BY MANIPULATING SUTURE
- Hold the suture near the swaged end
- Align by maneuvering the suture

- Alternatively, needle can be adjusted by holding the suture near the swaged end of the needle and maneuvering it till the needle is aligned perpendicular to the jaws (Figs 5.22 to 5.25). ▶

- For erecting the needle, a preferred method is to place the needle on the serosal surface of viscera, preferably stomach. Press the upper jaw of open needle holder over the needle. The needle will automatically erect into correct position for suturing (Figs 5.26 to 5.29). ▶

After the ideal position is reached, the grip on the needle is tightened to lock it into position.

NEEDLE ERECTION BY PRESSING OVER IT

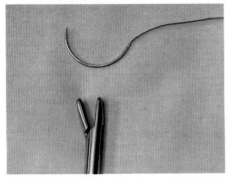

Fig. 5.26: Approach the needle with needle holder (inside abdomen the needle should be placed on the serosal surface of viscera, preferably stomach)

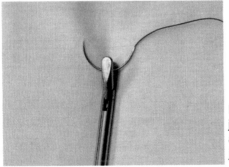

Fig. 5.27: Open the jaws of needle holder and place the upper jaw over the needle

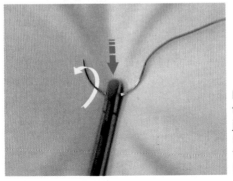

Fig. 5.28: Press over the needle with open jaws. Observe tshe needle getting erected. Grasp when properly aligned

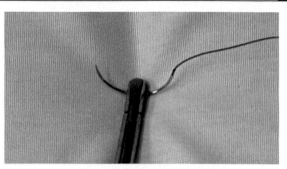

Fig. 5.29: **Well** aligned needle. Ready for suturing

NEEDLE ERECTION BY PRESSING OVER IT

- Place the needle on the serosal surface of viscera.
- Place the upper jaw of open needle holder over the needle and press down.
- Needle aligns with concavity upwards.
- Grip and start suturing (Fig. 5.30).

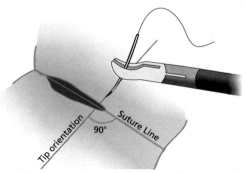

Fig. 5.30: The properly positioned needle is brought to the tissue defect, ready to begin the entrance bite

Driving the Needle

The plane of the needle should be perpendicular to the shaft of the instrument and the needle should be perpendicular to the suture line (Fig. 5.31).

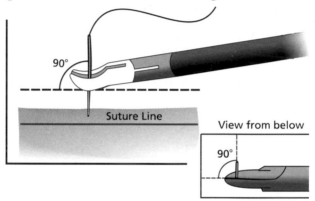

Fig. 5.31: Correct needle direction

- The needle tip should be rotated until it is perpendicular to the tissue, which is achieved by rotating the instrument counter-clockwise (Fig. 5.32). Needle insertion angle of 80°-100° is optimum for good suturing.[5]
- The needle is then hooked into the tissue at the entrance point and the precise alignment checked.
- If the surgeon is right handed, the needle is grasped in right instrument and driven across the tissue from right to left. Supination of the wrist will pass the needle clearly through the tissue without tearing (Fig. 5.33).

- If satisfactory, counter pressure is provided and the needle is slowly driven into the tissue, making sure that the direction of penetration is maintained head-on against tissue resistance (Fig. 5.34).
- Small adjustments can be made as necessary by pushing or pulling on the needle to alter its direction slightly.

Although this maneuver is quite challenging at first, it promotes good habits and self-confidence in precision control techniques.

CAUTION
- The fulcrum of needle holder is where it enters the abdominal wall and it is easy to traumatize the tissues by allowing too much torque at the end of needle holder.
- The surgeon should try to keep the path as short as possible.

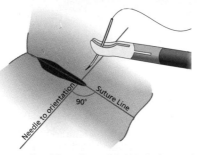

Fig. 5.32: The needle driver is to be rotated counter-clockwise in preparation for the entrance bite

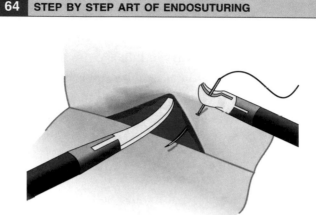

Fig. 5.33: The needle is positioned firmly in a needle driver, and countertraction is applied with the assisting grasper by lifting the tissue edge near the entrance point

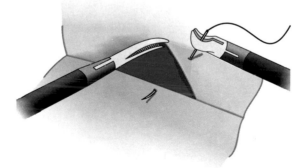

Fig. 5.34: For the exit bite, counterpressure is applied by gently lifting and folding back the corresponding tissue edge. In each case, the needle tip is driven head-on (perpendicular) against the tissue surface, requiring rotation of the needle driver, similar to a scooping motion

Selection of Entrance Point

When using a single armed needle the direction of the entrance bite from outside the tissue to inside is more difficult than an exit bite which is easier to perform where the needle passes from inside to outside. Therefore, in certain cases, double armed suturing is recommended because this is easier and safer.

- Select the first entrance point in a way to create a suture line ideal for reconstruction.
- Make it site dependent, e.g. Suturing the colon has critical concerns such as a water tight suture line and having inverted edges.
- Avoid making an entrance bite too small or too thick or a combination of the two, resulting in tortuous suture line.

Amount of Bite

The selection of the entrance and exit bites will determine the amount of the bite. The amount of the bite needs to be precisely calculated for each structure, keeping in mind the function and reconstructive goal.

- Too little a bite may not provide adequate seal or strength.
- Too large a bite will result in a bulky suture line, possibly narrowing the lumen of a conduit and perhaps causing tissue necrosis.

Exit Bite

The exit bite is easier to perform than the entrance bite, therefore double armed suturing is encouraged where two exit bites could complete the stitch. This is especially advantageous during the anastomosis of conduits.

- To locate the proper exit point, the needle is turned upward (external direction), creating an upward tenting of the tissue.
- The correct point is estimated and adjustments can be made here to correct for the thickness of the bite.
- The needle after being driven through can be regrasped further back and pushed forward.
- The tip can be grasped either with the assisting grasper or needle driver.
- Needle is pulled out carefully adjusting it to minimize trauma.

Everywhere is walking distance if you have the time.
—Steven Wright

REFERENCES

1. Emam TA, Hanna G, Cuschieri A. Ergonomic principles of task alignment, visual display, and direction of execution of laparoscopic bowel suturing. Surg Endosc 2002 Feb; 16(2): 267-71.

2. Frede T, Stock C, Renner C, Budair Z. Geometry of laparoscopic suturing and knotting techniques. J Endourol 1999 Apr; 13(3): 191-8.

3. Berguer R, Forkey DL, Smith WD. The effect of laparoscopic instrument working angle on surgeons' upper extremity workload. Surg Endosc 2001 Sep; 15(9):1027-9.

4. Emam TA, Hanna GB, Kimber C, et al. Effect of intra-corporeal-extracorporeal instrument length ratio on endoscopic task performance and surgeon movements. Arch Surg 2000 Jan; 135(1): 62-5; discussion 66.

5. Joice P, Hanna GB, Cuschieri A. Ergonomic evaluation of laparoscopic bowel suturing. Am J Surg 1998 Oct; 176(4): 373-8.

Chapter 6

Intracorporeal Suturing Techniques

- **LINEAR INCISIONS AND LACERATIONS**
  - **Tissue Factors**
  - **Suture Factors**
- **INTERRUPTED SUTURING**
- **CONTINUOUS SUTURING**
  - **Suture Material**
- **DUCTAL ANASTOMOSIS**
  - **End to End Anastomosis**
  - **End to Side Anastomosis**
  - **Side to Side Anastomosis**
- **TIPS**

Not everything that is more difficult is more meritorious.

—*Thomas Aquinas*

Knot tying and suturing as means to approximate tissue constitute the essence of surgical practice. These skills are basic to all operations and are among the first things learned by the medical student and surgical intern. All surgeons have practiced tying square knots with one or both hands and driving sutures through synthetic or preserved animal tissue.

Laparoscopic intracorporeal suturing is difficult, a complex task involving several integrated skills such as needle handling, suturing, and knotting.

Running suturing is even more complex in the closed environment secondary to the angles of the suture lines, the tension maintained on the suture line, and the need to secure the ends, including tying a knot from the tail of the suture to the loop of the preceding stitch.

When constructing suture lines, tissues should be prepared so that re-approximation can be accomplished with minimum tension.

Tissues can be positioned by the assistant or self retaining retractors.

LINEAR INCISIONS AND LACERATIONS

The intracorporeal suture line is composed of continuous, interrupted or a combination of both types of suturing. Factors need to be kept in mind before constructing a linear suture line. These factors are:

Tissue Factors

1. Length of incision
2. Type of tissue
3. Function of tissue

Suture Factors

Length of suture: The common mistake in suturing is to work with too long or too short a piece of suture. For a single stitch, the thread should be approximately 5½ inches long. A good rule of thumb for a running suture is to allow 5½ inches for the first stitch and ½ inch for each additional stitch. A suture : incision ratio of 9:1 is best for longer suture lines and 10:1 is better for short suture lines.[1]

INTERRUPTED SUTURING

• Interrupted sutures may be constructed using a suspension slip-knot technique, to approximate tissue that may be under tension, or where visibility is needed for placement of further sutures.

- Sutures should be placed evenly, bringing the tissues together without excessive tension or mis-alignment of layers.
- The number of stitches required is based on the number needed to complete a suture line adequately or provide tissue edge alignment.
- Intracorporeal suturing can be accomplished with one of the described methods. Extracorporeal (Roeder/Melzer/Duncan, etc) knots can be useful for the novice.
- More often used for colorectal anastomosis, closure of enterotomy or if an inadvertent intraperitoneal injury needs to be repaired.

CONTINUOUS SUTURING

- This is quicker but more difficult to perform correctly.
- This should be learnt after interrupted suturing, where hand to eye co-ordination, basic suturing and tissue alignment are picked up.
- For the ease of performance, continuous suturing requires three ports: two positioned such that the two needle holders meet along the line of intended anastomosis at right angles, and the third which is sited cephalad to the area, is used by the assistant to grasp the suture and take the slack after each needle passage.

- The continuous suturing technique begins and ends in an anchoring knot. The initial knot of the running suture can be formed by a standard square knot or a Jamming knot (described later).

- For the running portion of the suture, one may use simple over and over running suture or intermittent lock stitches to maintain tissue tension.

- It is important to have an assistant using a rubber shod grasping device to follow the suture and maintain tension over the closure. After each needle passage, the assistant picks up the slack and keep uniform tension on the suture line. This has the added advantage of tenting and stabilizing the tissues, thereby, facilitating needle passage.

- To finish the suture line, the suture must be fixed with another knot. This may be tied using a standard square knot or an Aberdeen knot.

- During training one should practice suturing in both directions. To and fro, left to right and right to left.

- Continuous suturing can be used to close mesenteric, intestinal or peritoneal defect or to accomplish colorectal anastomosis.

Suture Material

The choice of suture material is important. This is because different sutures behave differently.

- Stiff, springy monofilament sutures run in a non-interlocking fashion and promote speed, but may result in an uneven suture line, although it is still sometimes the material of choice.
- Woven threads, particularly 2-0 and 3-0 silk have a tendency to drag and lock the suture line and every such stitch has to be adjusted to the necessary tension.
- Use of single-armed suture is suitable for linear suture lines: however, double-armed or double-pointed needles can also be used.

DUCTAL ANASTOMOSIS

Laparoscopic ductal suturing is challenging but feasible. Ductal structures with less critical demanding technique (such as GI tract) can be accomplished with end to side, end to end and side to side techniques. The following are required:
- Watertight seal
- Proper mucosal approximation.

End to End Anastomosis

The preferred method for joining conduits of equal caliber and wall-thickness.
- The number of stitches and the amount of bite are estimated for each particular organ, depending on its function.

- Either interrupted or continuous sutures can be used. Interrupted stitches give greater precision and control; the continuous technique is more rapid, although less forgiving.
- Assisting devices such as self-retractors, clamps or intraluminal stents can be useful.

End to Side Anastomosis

Allows the union of conduits with disparate lumens and wall thickness.

- Is easier to accomplish than end to end anastomosis.
- It is less invasive than the end to end technique because the fenestration on the recipient structure involves only part of its circumference.
- Conduction of the luminal contents is a concern because it is necessary to turn a corner to advance.

Side to Side Anastomosis

It provides a convenient joining of conduits that normally lie side by side.

- Is similar to end to side anastomosis and is frequently employed in the gastrointestinal tract.

TIPS

Manipulation of bowel around fixed cannula positions require patience and care. While the instruments themselves may be atraumatic, as soon as the bowel is pulled or pushed, the apex of contact between the forceps and the bowel very easily acts as a point where perforation is induced. Steps to minimize this hazard include the following:

1. Before bowel manipulation, ensure it is free of adhesions and mobile.
2. Patient positioning and tilting of the operating table uses gravity to displace the bowel without the need for repeated manipulation.
3. Both of the operators' hands should be used to improve tactile feedback.
4. With the third grasper in the hands of the assistant, this allows a step-wise grasping and release of bowel to 'walk' along the bowel efficiently to the region of interest.
5. No hesitation should be felt about using a fifth access port if required.
6. The grasper must be kept in the field of view at all times while being moved to minimize the chance of bowel injury.
7. On occasion the telescope might better be inserted through one of the other ports as far away form the bowel as possible to provide a panoramic view of the proceedings.
   - The spring-handled atraumatic grasping forceps and Dorsey bowel grasper are the best instruments for bowel manipulation.

- Frequently the atraumatic graspers slip when excessive traction is applied, although at times irritating, it provides a safeguard against accidental bowel perforation.

- With due care, dissecting forceps may be useful to retract bowel when applied to the appendices epiploicae.

REFERENCE

1. Desai PJ, Moran ME, Calvano CJ. Running suturing: the ideal length facilitates this task. J Endourol 2000 Mar; 14(2): 191-4.

Chapter 7

Intracorporeal Knot Tying

- **TYPES OF INTRACORPOREAL SURGICAL KNOTS**
  - **Square Knot**
  - **Square Slip Knot**
  - **Ligature Slip Knot**
  - **Surgeon's Knot**
  - **Jamming Slip Knot** *(Starter Knot)*
  - **Aberdeen Knot** *(Terminal Knot)*
- **TECHNIQUE OF INTRACORPOREAL KNOTTING**
  - **The Suture**
  - **Selection of Suture Material**
  - **The Instruments**
  - **Creation of 'C' Loop**
  - **Wrapping**
  - **Tail Pick Up and Configuration of the Knot**
  - **Tightening and Completion of First Half Knot**
  - **Configuration of Subsequent Knots**
  - **Completion of Knot**
- **INTRACORPOREAL TWIST TECHNIQUE**
- **SQUARE SLIP KNOT**
- **KNOT SUBSTITUTES**
- **ERGONOMICS IN INTRACORPOREAL SUTURING**

"Dress me slowly, I am in hurry."
—*Napoleon Bonaparte*

Intracorporeal knot tying requires substantial practice for mastery and is a challenge for the novice. Advanced laparoscopic surgical techniques are hampered by the inability to perform intracorporeal knotting. This is an essential and fundamental skill because it is based on time honoured universally adaptable methods that can utilize readily available materials. Intracorporeal suturing is invaluable for a laparoscopic surgeon, not only because of its universal applicability but also because of tremendous cost benefits it carries. For instance, intracorporeal suturing of Mesh in hernia repair obviates the cost of tacker/stapler/anchoring device (10,000/- to 15,000/-!).

Internal knots are used in relation to suturing more commonly than external knots. Irrespective of the method used, the number and type of suture material used, internal knotting requires practice to be performed smoothly and quickly, and this is best achieved by use, by the practice bench with foam or animal tissue specimens.

Though taxing to learn and even more tedious to perform Intracorporeal suturing possesses specific advantages.

The advantages are:

- Diminished traffic of instruments and sutures through the ports.
- Decreased risk of infection because of lesser contamination of the internal environment.
- Lesser tissue trauma as compared to extracorporeal knots.

The **ideal knot** needs to be selected
1. Simple to tie.
2. Hold securely.
3. Be adaptable for multipurpose use.

Such a knot is the traditional 'Square-knot'. The added feature is that it can be converted to a 'Slip-knot' that is adjustable and re-convertible into the locking configuration (Square-knot) numerous times. This permits the employment of the Slip-knot suspension technique, a practical method of conduit anastomosis.

TYPES OF INTRACORPOREAL SURGICAL KNOTS

Square Knot (Fig. 7.1) ▶

Basic knot, essential for open and laparoscopic surgery. First single half knot is followed by another half knot in opposite direction. It is prone to slippage when the tissues are under tension. Must slippage occur, square knot can be converted to square slip knot and tightened.

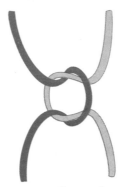

Fig. 7.1: Square knot

Square Slip Knot (Fig. 7.2)

Essentially it consists of traditional square knot composed of two half knots in opposing direction. After the square knot is configured, it is untumbled to achieve a slip knot configuration. The slip knot is put in place to achieve adequate tissue tension by sliding. It is further secured in place with the help of a third

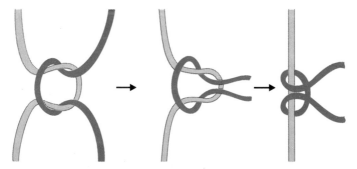

Fig. 7.2(a): Square knot   Fig. 7.2(b): Sliding configuration

half knot in opposite direction. It is ideal when the tissue edge distraction is encountered as in the repair of defects, *viz.* hiatal hernia. It works best with low friction suture material such as monofilament synthetic material.

Advantages

- Ability to secure the knot in difficult locations.
- The use of standard tying methods.
- Lack of extracorporeal knot creation or need for a pushing device.[1]

Ligature Slip Knot (Fig. 7.3)

It is similar to a square knot except that the first half knot is double instead of being single. Although it slides less readily than square knot, its holding strength is greater.

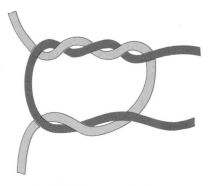

Fig. 7.3: Ligature slip knot

Surgeon's Knot (Fig. 7.4)

Similar to the traditional knot used in open surgery, once the tissue edges are approximated and held together with the first double half knot, the second and third opposing single half knots are tied. It is best configured in high friction material such as silk and braided synthetic material.

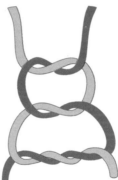

Fig. 7.4: Surgeon's knot

Jamming Slip Knot *(Starter Knot)*

When continuous suturing is to be accomplished the starter knot is generally configured externally with the help of Jamming slip knot (Figs 7.5 and 7.6). Once formed the knot is slipped from tail to form a 1 cm loop, after which the tail is cut short to 1.5 cm length. A suture with a Jamming knot at one end is introduced through the cannula. The needle is passed through the tissue until the loop impinges on the tissue (Fig. 7.7).

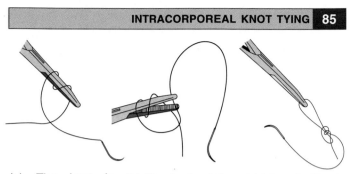

(a) The knot is started by wrapping the tail of the suture around a needle holder

(b) The body of the suture 5 cm from the loop is grasped with the tip of the needle holder

(c) It is pulled back through the initial wrap to create the loop

Fig. 7.5: Jamming slip knot (Starter knot)

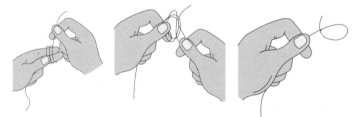

Fig. 7.6: Slip knot is made by manually encircling two fingers twice, then passing the thread through the double loop. The loops are pulled tight

The needle is reversed and is passed through the loop. The long suture is then grasped near the loop, and the tail is pulled in the opposite direction to slide the loop on the suture, Jamming the knot.

A Jamming loop knot made outside the abdomen facilitates the initiation of a running suture. It works well to start a running suture, as it obviates intra-corporeal knot tying.

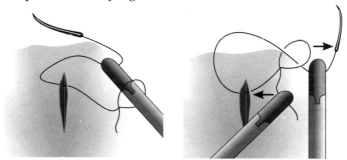

Fig. 7.7: The needle is passed through the loop. The long suture is held near the loop while the tail is held by other instrument. The two are pulled in opposite direction to slide the knot in place

This technique can also be used for interrupted suturing. In that case, the knot needs to be reinforced with a restraining hitch. Only one such hitch is necessary for silk, but other materials like polyamide, which do not lock as well as silk, require two restraining hitches.

Aberdeen Knot *(Terminal Knot)*

At completion of a running suture line, the tail may be secured to the last loop with an Aberdeen or Crotchet knot. After completing the running suture, the knot is begun bringing a loop of the free suture underneath the previous bite and tightening it by pulling on the

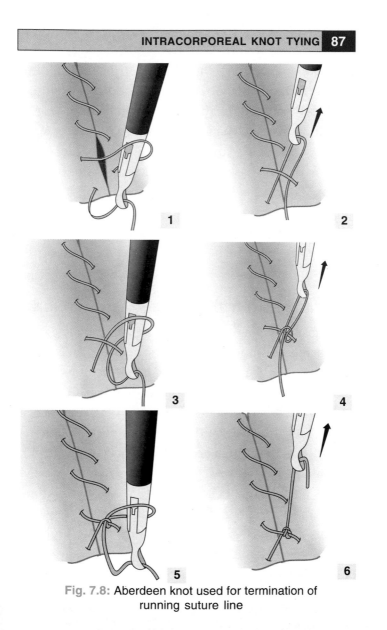

Fig. 7.8: Aberdeen knot used for termination of running suture line

attached end of the loop (Fig. 7.8). While holding tension in the first loop, a second loop of the suture body is then brought through the first loop, then a third loop through the second, and so on. Good team effort is necessary to master the knot because the surgeon and the assistant must keep tension on the suture. After three to five interlocking loops, depending on the knot strength of the suture material, the free end of the suture is introduced through the last loop before traction is applied close to the loop to secure the knot.

TECHNIQUE OF INTRACORPOREAL KNOTTING ▶

The basic movements of knot tying, after analysis can be assembled into a teachable sequence, choreographed into the least number of required movements and standardized for predictable results. The breakdown of movements also allows for the sequence to be recognizable, and permits slow meticulous execution in the limited access magnified surgical field.

The choreographed sequence presented in the figures must be practiced precisely to achieve the time and effort saving benefits of this approach.

This technique can be used to form various type of intracorporeal knots, *viz.* square, square slip, surgeon's or ligature knot, etc.

The Suture

The length of suture is critical to good suturing. Too long a suture makes the procedure tiring and clumsy in order to trace the tail. For a single stitch, the thread should be approximately 5½ inches long. A good rule of thumb for a running suture is to allow 5½ inches for the first stitch and ½ inch for each additional stitch. Incision : suture length of 1:9 for short incisions and 1:10 for longer incisions is optimum.[2]

For better understanding, we can divide the suture in two parts. Once the needle is pushed across the tissues which need to be approximated, the suture can be viewed as having two parts. The part towards the needle is longer and is referred to as the standing part. Contralateral part, i.e. towards the tail end is shorter.

Selection of Suture Material

Selection of suture material is critical. The ability to use instruments to handle suture material with memory and elastic deformation characteristics is essential.

- Stiff, thick monofilament suture is difficult to use because it bends and springs unpredictably, does not deform to lock the knot in place and requires multiple hitches to secure.

- On the other hand of the spectrum is a flimsy braided suture that becomes limp in the surgical field, shreds when grasped and when pulled harder, it locks irreversibly.

- Braided polyfilament sutures (absorbable or silk 2-0 and 3-0) are more compliant and convenient for intracorporeal suturing.

The Instruments

Atleast one needle driver/holder is needed for driving the needle inside the tissues. The other instrument is the assisting instrument and can be another needle holder or simply a grasper. It is needed for stabilizing the tissues, needle or the suture during suturing.

Creation of 'C' Loop (Figs 7.9 to 7.11)

The long end of the suture is to be fashioned in the form of 'C' shape. It is formed on the side opposite to the tail of the suture. If the tail is on the right side then right (R) instrument is used for holding the long end of the suture and the C loop is formed on the left side. The left (L) instrument will hence be used in wrapping. The idea of creating the C loop is to have a shoulder around which wrapping can be done.

Wrapping (Figs 7.12 to 7.17)

Wrapping entails winding the C loop around the contralateral instrument. It can be done in two ways:
- Twirling the instrument around the thread held by the needle holder.
- Wrapping the thread around the instrument which is held stationary.

- Although wrapping is better to twirling, generally a combination of varying degrees of both is used.

TIPS
- Always keep the needle under view.
- The suture must be short (not exceeding 5 inches in length).
- If the C loop can be made to stand up in front of the camera, the wrapping and knotting can be done conveniently and rapidly.
- Following wrapping, the tail must be grasped as near the tip as possible.
- For secure knotting, the wrapping of the second component of the knot must be in the reverse direction to the first and the third component identical to the first.
- Close camera work aids in depth perception.

Tail Pick Up and Configuration of the Knot

Once wrapping is completed, the assistant holder (used for wrapping) is advanced to pick the tail of the suture (Figs 7.18 and 7.19). The wraps are spilled over the tip of the assisting instrument and the tail, forming the start of the first half knot (Figs 7.20 and 7.21).

Tightening and Completion of First Half Knot

The assisting and the active instruments while holding the tail and the standing part of suture respectively, are pulled in opposite direction, hence tightening the knot (Fig. 7.22). The tail end is kept stationary while maintaining the tug, and standing part is pulled in opposite direction.

CAUTION
1. *'If you pull the tail, you are in the jail.'* During tightening, the tail end is kept stationary and under tension towards opposite side, while the standing part is moved to the other side. Do not pull the tail end.
2. Do not pull very strongly. It can strangulate the tissue or the sutures can cut through.
3. While pulling make sure the instruments are under view. Inadvertent injury can occur at this stage.

Configuration of Subsequent Knots

Similar technique as used for the first half knot is utilized. The C loop is, however, formed on the opposite side (Figs 7.23 and 7.24). If the initial C loop was on left side then the current (second) C (or 'D') loop would be on the right side. Hence, L instrument would be used for holding the suture, whereas R instrument would be used for wrapping (Figs 7.25 to 7.31). More C loops are formed on opposite sides as required for a particular knot.

TECHNIQUE OF INTRACORPOREAL KNOTTING: CREATION OF C LOOP

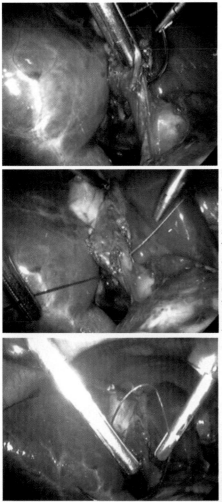

Fig. 7.9: Transfixation of structure which needs to be ligated

Fig. 7.10: Right (R) and left (L) instruments holding the right and left limbs of suture; Right being the tail (shorter) end and left being the longer (standing) part of suture. Never hold the suture by needle unless driving it into tissues!

Fig. 7.11: Fashion the longer part of the suture (standing part) in the form of a C shape, known as C loop, on the side opposite to the tail (i.e. left side)

TECHNIQUE OF INTRACORPOREAL KNOTTING:
WRAPPING

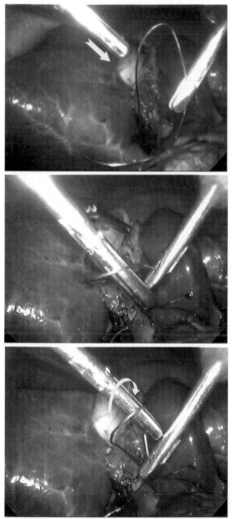

Fig. 7.12: Continue to hold with R instrument, while advancing L instrument over the C loop

Fig. 7.13: Advance and place the L instrument over the C loop

Fig. 7.14: Using wrapping motion of L instrument, begin forming wraps of the C loop

TECHNIQUE OF INTRACORPOREAL KNOTTING: WRAPPING

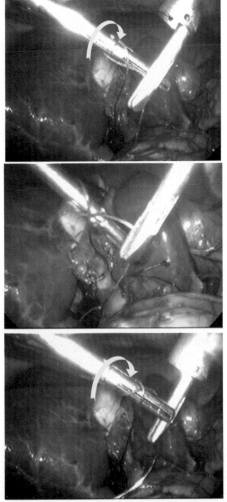

Fig. 7.15: Continue wrapping movement to fashion first wrap (throw) of the C loop

Fig. 7.16: First wrap (throw) completed

Fig. 7.17: In order to form a surgeons knot, continue the wrapping movement to further fashion second wrap

TECHNIQUE OF INTRACORPOREAL KNOTTING: TAIL PICK UP

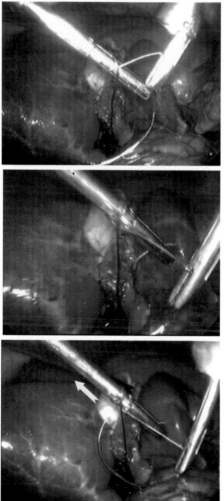

Fig. 7.18: Once the second wrap is complete, advance both instruments towards the tail end of the suture

Fig. 7.19: Tail pick up: With the help of L instrument catch hold of the tip of tail

Fig. 7.20: Withdraw the L instrument while keeping the R instrument firm and stationary, in order to spill the wraps over the tip and the tail

TECHNIQUE OF INTRACORPOREAL KNOTTING: TIGHTENING

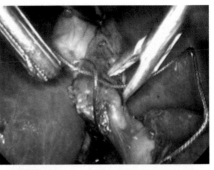

Fig. 7.21: Wraps spilled over the tail and the tip of the L instrument configuring the first double half knot

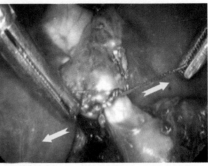

Fig. 7.22: Pull the instruments in the opposite direction tightening the first double half knot. (Keep the instruments under view while pulling). The first half knot is hence completed

TECHNIQUE OF INTRACORPOREAL KNOT TYING

- Create C loop on left side
- Wrapping (two wraps for surgeon's knot) by left instrument
- Tail pick up
- Spill the wraps by withdrawing left instrument
- Tighten by pulling instruments in opposite direction

TECHNIQUE OF INTRACORPOREAL KNOTTING CREATION OF 'C' LOOP ON CONTRALATERAL SIDE

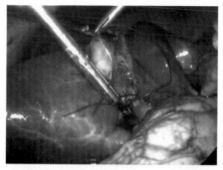

Fig. 7.23: Formation of C loop on the contra-lateral side (right side). Using the L instrument to hold the longer part of (standing part) suture, a C loop is fashioned on the right side

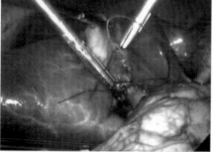

Fig. 7.24: The R instrument is kept over the C loop for wrapping

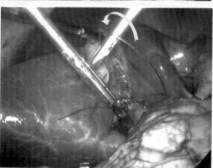

Fig. 7.25: Beginning of wrapping on same side

TECHNIQUE OF INTRACORPOREAL KNOTTING: WRAPPING

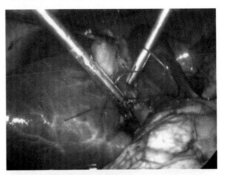

Fig. 7.26: Wrap (single) complete

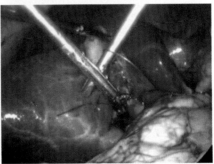

Fig. 7.27: Advance both instruments towards the tail

TECHNIQUE OF INTRACORPOREAL KNOT TYING
- Create C loop on right side
- Wrapping (single wrap) by right instrument
- Tail pick up
- Spill the wraps by withdrawing right instrument
- Tighten by pulling instruments in opposite direction

TECHNIQUE OF INTRACORPOREAL KNOTTING
TAIL PICK UP AND TIGHTENING

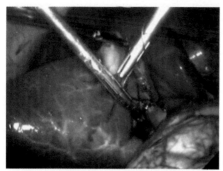

Fig. 7.28: Tail pick up

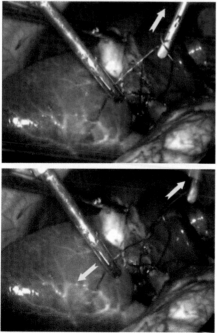

Fig. 7.29: Spill the wraps over the tail and the tip of instrument

Fig. 7.30: Distract the instruments in opposite direction

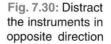

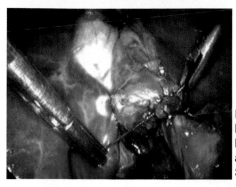

Fig. 7.31: Second half knot complete. Third half knot should be added to complete Surgeon's knot

Completion of Knot

Upon completion, endoscissors is brought into the field and the sutures are cut at an appropriate distant from the knot (1 cm for braided sutures). Extrasuture is removed from the field unless subsequent suturing is intended.

"Perfect practice makes practice perfect"

INTRACORPOREAL TWIST TECHNIQUE

This technique greatly simplifies the intracorporeal suturing. It is universally applicable for all suture sizes and is designed to consistently form a Surgeon's knot with minimal slippage. One end of the suture is rotated up the 5 mm grasper until three or four loops are formed (Fig. 7.32(1),(2)). A second grasper removes

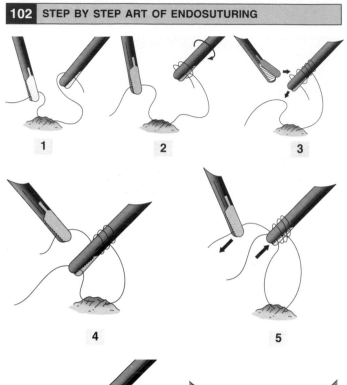

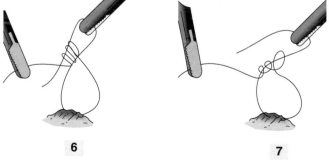

Fig. 7.32 (1 to 7): Intracorporeal twist technique

the suture end from the jaws of the rotating grasper and slides the end upward along the shaft (Fig. 7.32(3)). The other free suture end is grasped with the first grasper (Fig. 7.32(4)). As both instruments are pulled in opposite direction, a square knot is formed (Fig. 7.32(5)). The knot can be tightened against the tissue surface and will not loosen if a second knot is similarly fashioned and positioned on to the tissues (Fig. 7.32(6),(7)).

SQUARE SLIP KNOT 🔘

- The square knot is completed using the C loop technique as above (Figs 7.33 and 7.34).
- Catch the tail end and the suture loop on the same side (Fig. 7.35). The two instruments (while holding the tail end and the suture loop of the same side) are distracted in a vertical plane (Fig. 7.36).
- The square knot gets converted to a slip knot and its appearance visibly changes (Fig. 7.36).

CAUTION
The initial square knot should not be extremely tight otherwise, conversion to slip configuration may not be possible.

- While continuing to hold at the tail of the suture, the instrument holding the suture loop is released and is now used to stradle the suture just proximal to the knot (Fig. 7.37).

SQUARE SLIP KNOT: STEPS

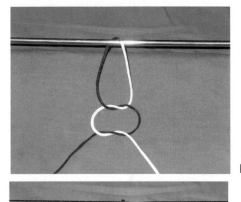

Fig. 7.33: Square knot configuration

Fig. 7.34: Square knot tightened

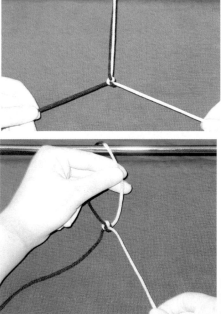

Fig. 7.35: Hold the loop and the tail end of the same side

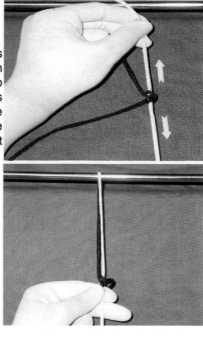

Fig. 7.36: Pull the hands in opposite direction while holding on the loop and the tail end, thus putting the white suture under tension. (Observe the change in knot configuration!)

Fig. 7.37: Continue to hold with your right hand and use the index and the thumb of the left hand (respective laparoscopic instruments during surgery) to slide the knot

SQUARE SLIP KNOT
- Tie a square knot
- Distract the tail end and the loop of the same side
- Conversion to slipping configuration occurs
- Slide the knot to destination
- Pull the ends in opposite direction
- Conversion to square knot occurs
- Secure with another half knot

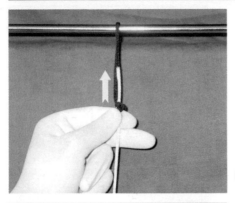

Fig. 7.38: Slide the knot in place

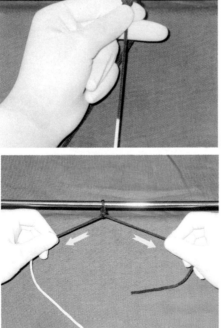

Fig. 7.39: Square slip knot slid to destination

Fig. 7.40: Pull the ends in opposite direction to reconvert to square knot. This can be secured with another half knot

- By applying countertraction at the tail end of the suture the knot is milked up to achieve the desired amount of tension and approximation of the tissues (Fig. 7.39).

- Reconversion to square knot occurs when the instruments apply traction in opposite direction at the tail end and the standing part of suture (Fig. 7.40).

- Further security is added by throwing another half knot in opposite direction as described previously using the C loop technique.

KNOT SUBSTITUTES

It is possible to replace external knots with knot clips. The **Lapraty knot clip** (Ethicon Endosurgery Inc.) is made of bioabsorbable, polydiaxonone suture and can therefore, be used in various situations, but it does involve additional costs. The friction of the Lapraty is only suitable when pressed on size 3-0 polyfilament thread; it is useful to start and end a running suture. These knot clips are useful for placing the first suture to take the tension of the tissue for the subsequent knots. Some surgeons use these for placing the first suture during a laparoscopic Nissen fundoplication.

Another knot substitute has been described by Buess in Germany for the use during endocavitary rectal suturing. In this technique, compressible **silver**

beads are applied to the suture and compressed in place at the desired point of the suture's tail, similar to applying shot weights to the fishing line.

ERGONOMICS IN INTRACORPOREAL SUTURING

- Good magnifiction.
- Economy of movements.
- Directional hold principle.
- Avoid instrument cross over.
- Correct choreographed knot tying.
- Knots on the surface of tissue.
- Close instrument jaws except during grasping.
- Apply knots close to the tail.
- Keep instruments under view.

But in science, the credit goes to the man who convinces the world, not to whom it first occurs.

—*Osler*

REFERENCES

1. Meng MV, Stoller ML. Laparoscopic intracorporeal square-to-slip knot. Urology 2002 Jun; 59(6): 932-3.
2. Desai PJ, Moran ME, Calvano CJ. Running suturing: the ideal length facilitates this task. J Endourol 2000 Mar; 14(2): 191-4.

Chapter 8

Extracorporeal Knot Tying

- **TECHNIQUE OF SUTURING USING EXTRACORPOREAL KNOTS**
- **TYPES OF EXTRACORPOREAL KNOTS**
  - **Roeder Knot**
  - **Melzer Knot**
  - **Texas Endosurgery Knot**
  - **Duncan Slip Knot**
  - **Tayside Knot**
  - **The Indian Rope Trick**
- **DRAWBACKS OF EXTRACORPOREAL KNOTTING**

A knot is perfect or hopelessly wrong.

—*Ashley*

Safe reliable knotting is crucial to tissue approximation. In laparoscopic surgery special techniques are required to achieve this purpose. Both internal and external knotting is possible after the acquisition of the necessary skills, which can only be obtained by practice on the bench trainer. Many surgeons who have recently taken up laparoscopic surgery rely exclusively on clipping to secure ductal structures and vessels. This is an unsatisfactory practice since situations are often encountered when it is not possible to clip a structure safely, either because it is too large or because the access is limited. In other circumstances, the use of metal clips may be undesirable because of long-term consequences such as the internalization of a metal clip used to secure the cystic duct during cholecystectomy. In time, this may lead to the formation of ductal calculi.

Extracorporeal knotting is especially useful because it is similar to knots formed in open surgery. Following applications are useful:

1. In continuity ligature of ductal structures.
2. Approximating tissues under tension where an intracorporeal knot might slip before it could be adequately locked.

3. Used by the novice who has not achieved the necessary skills for intracorporeal knotting.
4. Suturing in case of limited access, where adequate space for intracorporeal maneouvering of suture is not available.

Advantages

1. Convenient to know.
2. Valuable for application of gut ligatures.
3. Can be used for configuring of pretied loops.

The simplest extracorporeal knot is the Roeder knot. It is also available in a pretied form. The pre-looped intracorporeal knot allies the sophistication of intracorporeal knot tying to the easiness and simplicity of the extracorporeal classic suturing. It renders intracorporeal knotting an easy and rapid task to achieve.[1]

TECHNIQUE OF SUTURING USING EXTRACORPOREAL KNOTS

- The technique involves the use of a long (90 cm) suture, which is passed down a 5 or 10 mm port.
- If the goal is suturing, the needle mounted on the end of the long suture is passed through tissue and brought out of the same port [Fig. 8.1(A)].
- If the goal is to ligate in continuity, the suture is passed around the structure to be ligated and again pulled out through the same port and exteriorized.

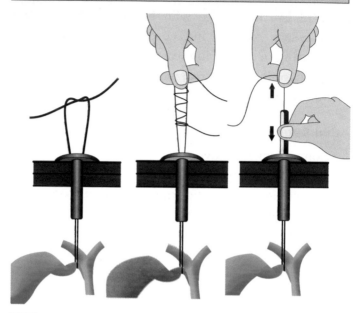

(A) The suture is passed around the structure which needs to be ligated, and drawn through the same port.

(B) An extracorporeal knot is configured.

(C) The knot is slid down with a plastic knot pusher to its destination. More throws can be similarly formed.

Fig. 8.1: Ligation in continuity using extracorporeal knot

- The suture is contained within the suture applicator or the reducer sheath to avoid entrapment within the trumpet or the flapper valve of the trocar. The assistant prevents the leakage by placing a finger over the exit site of the suture.

- To prevent scissoring effect of the suture over the structure around which it is passed, an instrument (needle holder/grasper) is inserted in the loop to take the tension and friction off the structure.
- Extracorporeal knot is created and a knot pushing instrument is placed over the knot [Fig. 8.1(B)].
- Even counter traction is placed on both ends of the suture and the knot is pushed down through the trocar until it is snug around the structure to be ligated.
- The knot pusher is then pulled out [Fig. 8.1(C)].
- A second throw is formed (reversed to the first throw if a square knot is desired).
- This knot is then pushed down with the knot pusher in an identical fashion.
- As many throws as are necessary, depending on the suture material are applied.
- A scissors is brought down along the suture or through another port to cut the suture material.

This technique works well for closing perforations of the gallbladder wall, for closure of a large cystic duct, and for ligating the base of the appendix.

TYPES OF EXTRACORPOREAL KNOTS

A variety of knots are available. Each has its own unique technique of configuration and specific application. Knots in which the second throw contains two or more turns are most secure.[2]

Roeder Knot (Figs 8.3 to 8.23) ▶
(Aide memoire 1-3-1)

The knot was described by Roeder in 1918 for tonsillectomy and introduced in Laparoscopic surgery by Semm. The knot is well known and used for construction of pre-formed catgut loops. It works well only with catgut and to a lesser extent with silk. The safety of this knot improves six-fold after hydration due to swelling. The knot is acceptably safe when tied with silk as the material also swells with hydration.

Essential steps include:
- Initial half knot [Fig. 8.2(1)].
- Three and a half round turns over the limbs of the loop [Fig. 8.2(2)].
- Second half knot [Fig. 8.2(3)].
- Careful stacking of turns between first and second half knots by gentle pulling on the tail and digital pressure on the standing part of the suture [Fig. 8.2(4)].
- Excess tail is cut off.
- Sliding the knot down to its position.
- The knot slides down with relative ease and locks by traction aginst pushing rod.

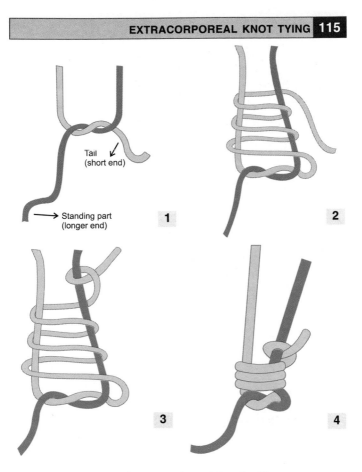

Tail
(short end)

Standing part
(longer end)

Fig. 8.2: Configuration of Roeder Knot

ROEDER KNOT: STEPS

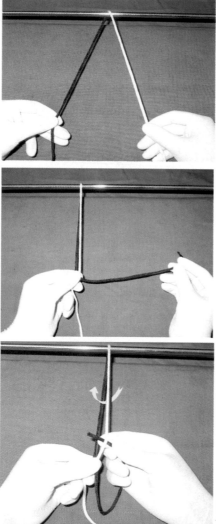

Fig. 8.3: Black (B) left and white (W) right sutures for configuring Roeder knot

Fig. 8.4: (B) Left suture is passed over right (W) suture

Fig. 8.5: First half knot made by hooking the left (B) limb from under the right (W) limb

ROEDER KNOT: STEPS

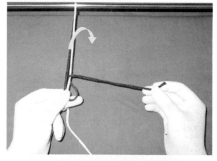

Fig. 8.6: First half knot completion by passing over the right (W) limb

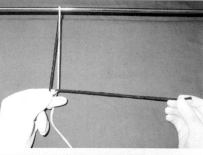

Fig. 8.7: Half knot completed by pulling the tail

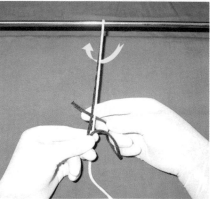

Fig. 8.8: First turn made by passing the tail end beneath both the limbs

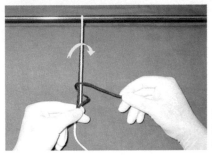

Fig. 8.9: First turn being accomplished by turning around both the limbs

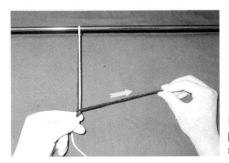

Fig. 8.10: First turn completed by pulling the tail snug fit

ROEDER KNOT: STEPS
- Aide-memoire: 1-3-1
- First half knot (around single R limb)
- Three turns (around both the limbs)
- Second half knot (around single R limb)

ROEDER KNOT: STEPS

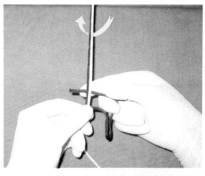

Fig. 8.11: Second turn begun by passing the tail end beneath both the limbs

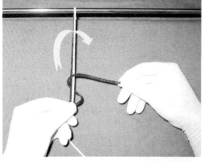

Fig. 8.12: Second turn accomplished by turning the tail end around both the limbs

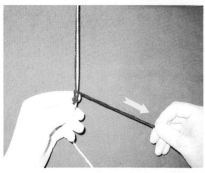

Fig. 8.13: Second turn completed by pulling the tail end

ROEDER KNOT: STEPS

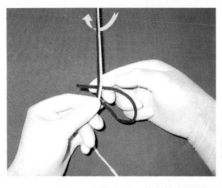

Fig. 8.14: Third turn (same as Ist and IInd) begun by passing the tail end under both the limbs

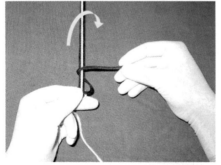

Fig. 8.15: Third turn formed by turning around both the limbs

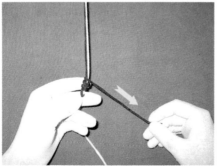

Fig. 8.16: Third turn completed by pulling the tail adequately to tighten the turn

ROEDER KNOT: STEPS

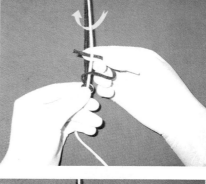

Fig. 8.17: Second half knot begun by passing the tail beneath the Right (W) limb

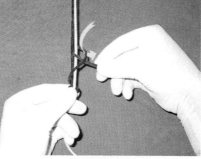

Fig. 8.18: Second half knot progressed by passing the tail in the loop formed by the black (B) suture

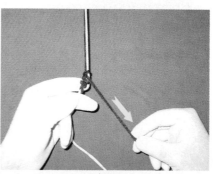

Fig. 8.19: Second half knot completed by pulling the tail to snuggly fit the knot

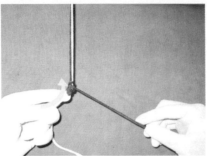

Fig. 8.20: Stacking of turns between knots with forefinger of left hand while tail is under gentle traction

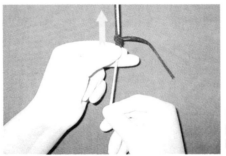

Fig. 8.21: Roeder knot is now ready to be slid into position

ROEDER KNOT: STEPS

- Aide-memoire: 1-3-1
- First half knot (around single R limb)
- Three turns (around both the limbs)
- Second half knot (around single R limb)

ROEDER KNOT: STEPS

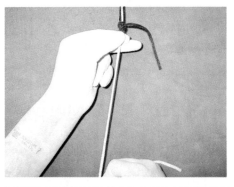

Fig. 8.22: Slide the knot between thumb and forefinger (knot pusher during surgery) by keeping the suture under gentle traction

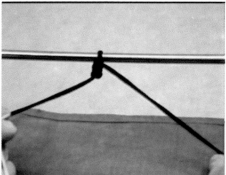

Fig. 8.23: Roeder knot completed and tightened over the target

`Melzer Knot ▶
(Figs 8.25-8.53)
(Aide memoire 2-3-2)

This is a modification of Roeder knot and was introduced by Melzer in 1991, Tubingen, Germany. It is much stronger then original Roeder knot and was developed for PDS (Polydioxonone). Chances of spontaneous loosening are less. However, with catgut the sliding is not smooth but much restricted.

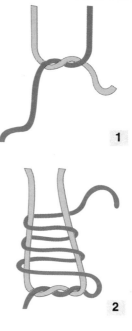

Essential steps include:

* Double initial half knot [Fig. 8.24(1)].
* Three and a half round turns over the limbs of the loop [Fig. 8.24(2)].
* Double second half knot [Fig. 8.24(3)].
* Careful stacking of turns between the knots.
* Sliding in position by push rod.

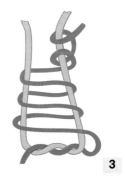

Fig. 8.24(1 to 3): Melzer knot

MELZER KNOT: STEPS

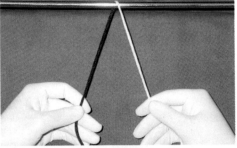

Fig. 8.25: Left (black) and right (white) limbs of suture for tying Melzer knot

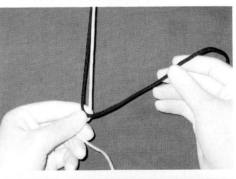

Fig. 8.26: Left (B) loop is brought over the right (W) limb

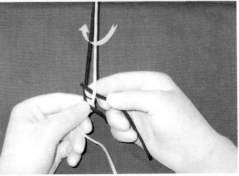

Fig. 8.27: First half knot made by hooking the left (B) limb from under the right (W) limb

MELZER KNOT: STEPS

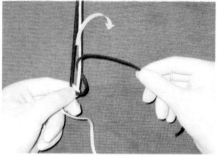

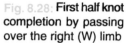
Fig. 8.28: **First half knot completion by passing over the right (W) limb**

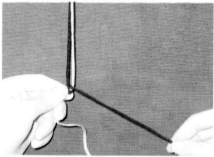

Fig. 8.29: **First half knot completed by pulling the tail**

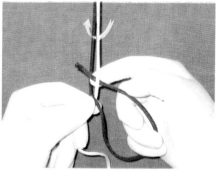

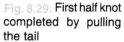
Fig. 8.30: **First double half knot begun by passing the tail under the right limb**

MELZER KNOT: STEPS

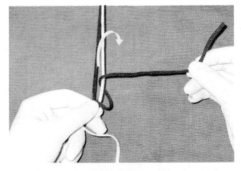

Fig. 8.31: First double half knot in progress by pulling the tail to the right

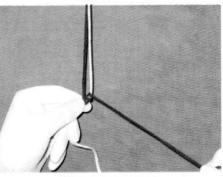

Fig. 8.32: First double half knot complete

MELZER KNOT: STEPS

- Aide-memoire: 2-3-2
- Two half knots (around single R limb)
- Three turns (around both the limbs)
- Two half knots (around single R limb)

MELZER KNOT: STEPS

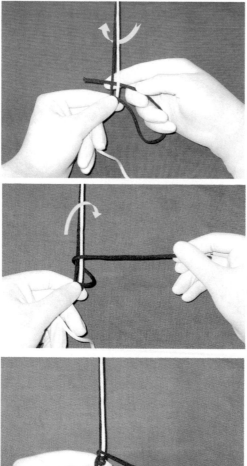

Fig. 8.33: First turn made by passing the tail end beneath both the limbs

Fig. 8.34: First turn being accomplished by turning around both the limbs

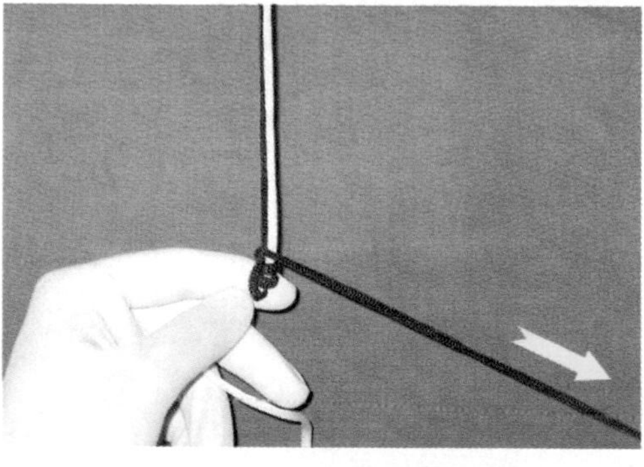

Fig. 8.35: First turn completed by pulling the tail snug fit

MELZER KNOT: STEPS

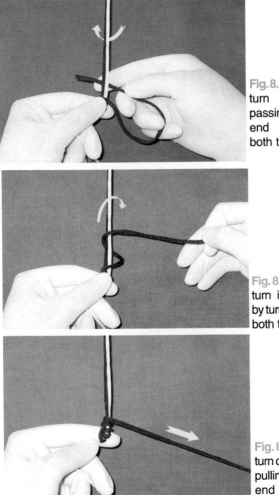

Fig. 8.36: Second turn begun by passing the tail end beneath both the limbs

Fig. 8.37: Second turn in progress by turning around both the limbs

Fig. 8.38: Second turn completed by pulling the tail end

MELZER KNOT: STEPS

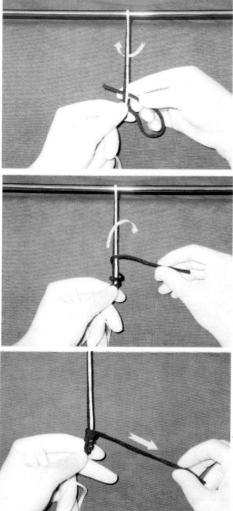

Fig. 8.39: Third turn (similar to Ist and IInd) begun by passing the tail end beneath both the limbs

Fig. 8.40: Third turn accomplished by turning the tail end around both the limbs

Fig. 8.41: Third turn completed by pulling the tail end

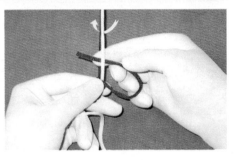

Fig. 8.42: Second half knot begun by passing the tail beneath the right (W) limb

MELZER KNOT: STEPS
- Aide-memoire: 2-3-2
- Two half knots (around single R limb)
- Three turns (around both the limbs)
- Two half knot (around single R limb)

With regards to excellence, it is not enough to know, but we must try to have and use it.

—Aristotle

MELZER KNOT: STEPS

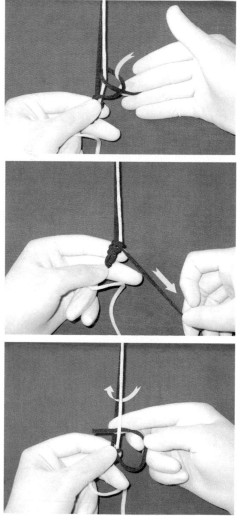

Fig. 8.43: Second half knot in progress, by passing the tail in the loop formed by the black suture

Fig. 8.44: Second half knot completed by pulling the tail to snuggly fit the knot

Fig. 8.45: Second double half knot begun similarly by passing the tail beneath the right (W) limb

MELZER KNOT: STEPS

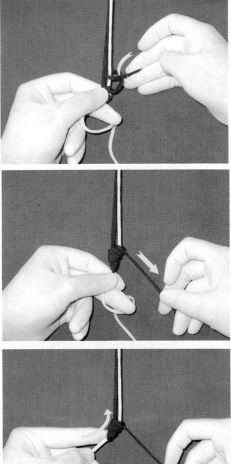

Fig. 8.46: Second double half knot in progress, by passing tail in the loop formed by the black suture

Fig. 8.47: Double half knot completed by pulling the tail to snuggly fit the knot

Fig. 8.48: Stacking of turns between knots with forefinger of left hand while tail is under gentle traction

MELZER KNOT: STEPS

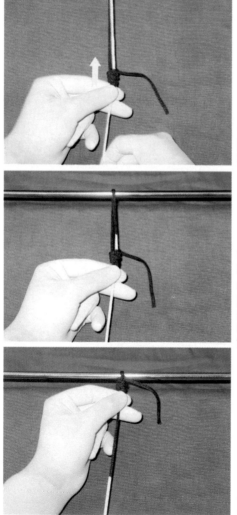

Fig. 8.49: Melzer knot is now ready to be slid into position

Fig. 8.50: Slide the knot between thumb and forefinger (knot pusher during surgery) by keeping the suture under gentle traction

Fig. 8.51: Knot tightened around the target destination

MELZER KNOT: STEPS

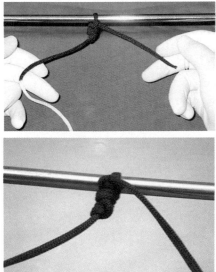

Fig. 8.52: Melzer knot completed and tightened over the target

Fig. 8.53: Melzer knot

Age cannot wither her,
nor custom stale her infinite variety.
    —*Anthony and Cleopatra. William Shakespeare*

Texas Endosurgery Institute Knot (TEI knot)

The Texas Endosurgery Institute knot can be tied in several ways, is somewhat difficult to tie, but may be useful for slicker materials, such as PDS (Fig. 8.54).

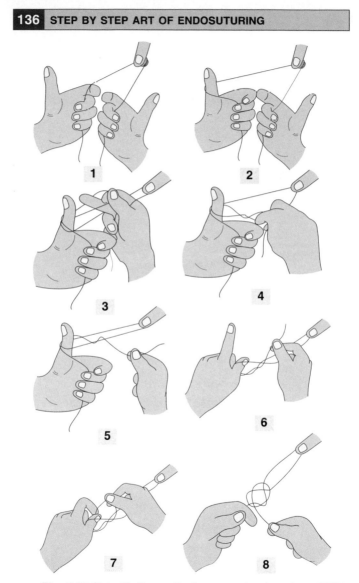

Fig. 8.54 (1 to 8): Texas Endosurgery Institute knot (TEI knot)

Duncan Slip Knot

Another alternative to Roeder knot is the knot, which is less prone to slippage as a result of the inherent design (Fig. 8.55). The slipping strength can further be increased if a simple half hitch is added to the knot after it has been down to the tissues and tightened. The half hitch provides additional safety and requires only a little more time.

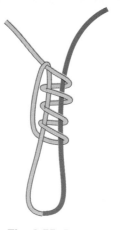

Fig. 8.55: Duncan slip knot

Tayside Knot

This knot is inspired by *Fisherman's* utility knot (Fig. 8.56) popular amongst the east coast of Scotland.

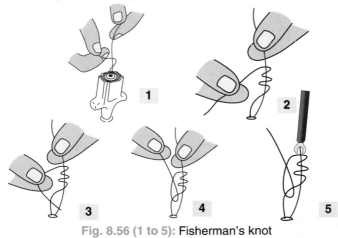

Fig. 8.56 (1 to 5): Fisherman's knot

Essential steps of **Tayside knot** include:
- Initial half knot [Fig. 8.57(1)].
- Four and half turns behind the half knot over the standing part [Fig. 8.57(2)].
- Creation of third loop by passing the tail through the second loop [Fig. 8.57(3)].
- The tail is passed through the second loop and under the third loop [Fig. 8.57(4)].

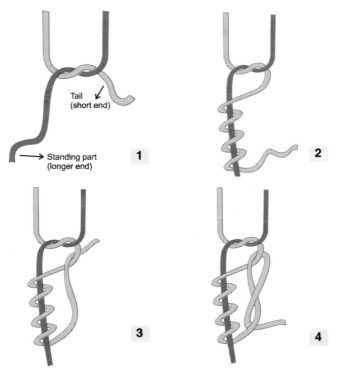

Fig. 8.57 (1 to 4): Configuration of Tayside knot

- The tail is pulled while the first half knot is pushed up by a finger inserted inside the noose to shape the knot.

The Indian Rope Trick

Laparoscopic suturing and knot tying require a lot of patience and practice and can be difficult, time consuming, and frustrating in spite of the advances made in the fields of instrumentation, optics, and imaging. A new technique has been described where an effort is made to make the procedure simpler by providing extracorporeal control of one limb of the suture. It involves percutaneous placement of the needle end of the suture in the abdomen and its removal using a modified 10 cm long cloth-sewing needle. The part of the suture hanging from the abdominal wall helps in the formation and the tying of both the extracorporeal and the intracorporeal knots. The extracorporeal knot is just pulled in percutaneously to make it intracorporeal and can be tightened easily without a knot pusher. The loop for making the intracorporeal knot is formed in one of the ways, and the half hitch or the surgeon's knot can be tightened by pulling one end extracorporeally and the other intracorporeally. Compared with the conventional method of laparoscopic suturing and knot tying, it was found to be easier to learn.[3]

DRAWBACKS OF EXTRACORPOREAL KNOTTING

1. It is liable to cause tissue trauma:
   - When large amount of suture is pulled through the needle tract.
   - When suture is pulled around a delicate tract.
   - Weight of the trocar creating torque on the suture, causing further tissue trauma.
2. Suture can get fractured by some knot pushers.
3. Low volume air-leak caused by suture through the trocar.
4. The knotpusher may become dislodged from the suture during transit into the abdominal cavity.
5. Some sutures don't slide well. (Monofilament, synthetic material slide better).
6. It requires close cooperation between surgeon and the assistant, which may become tedious and time consuming.

If you can describe clearly, without a diagram the precise technique of tying this / that knot, then you are the master of English tongue. —*Belloc*

REFERENCES

1. Nouira Y, Horchani A. The pre-looped intracorporeal knot: a new technique for knot tying in laparoscopic surgery. J Urol 2001 Jul; 166(1): 195-7.
2. Dinsmore RC. Laparoscopic intracorporeal square-to-slip knot. J Am Coll Surg. 1995 Jun; 180(6): 689-9.
3. Gaur DD. Laparoscopic suturing and knot tying: the Indian rope trick. J Endourol. 1998 Feb; 12(1): 61-6.

Chapter 9

Common Errors and Remedies

- **LOOSENING OF KNOT**
- **UNRAVELING OF KNOT**
- **SHORT SUTURE LENGTH**
  - **Half Moon Effect**
- **INCORRECT LOOP FORMATION**
  - **'S' Loop Formation**
  - **Reversed 'S' Loop**
  - **'O' Loop**
- **CROSSING INSTRUMENTS**
- **NEEDLE DEFLECTION AND REMEDY**
  - **Cause**
  - **Solution**
- **COMPLICATIONS OF SUTURING**

Experience is the name everyone gives to their mistakes
—*Lady Windermine, Oscar Wilde*

LOOSENING OF KNOT

When the first half knot is placed with the tissue edges pulled together in the correct position the resulting approximation should hold until the second half knot is configured and cinched down on top of the first. If the first half knot loosens during the time second knot is being completed the phenomenon is known as loosening (Fig. 9.1).

Knot loosening depends on the following factors:
- Skilled instrument maneuvering.
- *Selection of suturing material:* Braided materials have lesser tendency to loosen as compared to monofilament.
- *Selection of knotting technique:* Square knot loosens more often than surgeon's knot.

Remedy

1. Conversion to square slip knot configuration. ▶
2. Tightening the first half knot while the second half knot is being configured in the following way: ▶
   - Wrap the second half knot over the instrument (Fig. 9.2).
   - Pick the tail of the suture (Fig. 9.2).

CORRECTION OF LOOSENING OF FIRST HALF KNOT

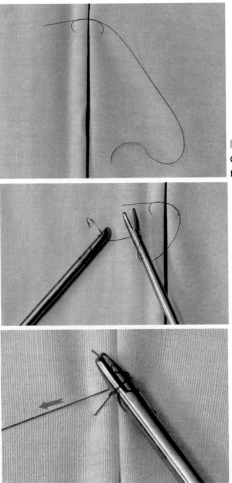

Fig. 9.1: Loosening of first half knot (common problem)

Fig. 9.2: Follow the steps for second half knot. Wrapping and tail pick-up shown here

Fig. 9.3: Without spilling the wraps continue to pull the L instrument maintaining traction on suture

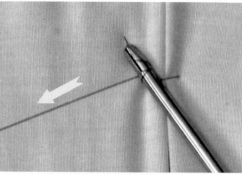

Fig. 9.4: Observe the first half knot getting tightened. Apply traction adequate for tightening the first half knot

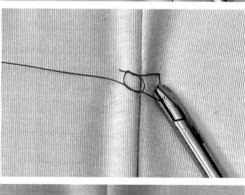

Fig. 9.5: Adequate level of tightness of first half knot reached. Spill the wrap of second half knot over the tip of assisting instrument

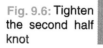

Fig. 9.6: Tighten the second half knot

- Do not spill the wrap over the tip at this stage (Fig. 9.3).
- Continue to tighten with the wraps over the assisting instrument without spilling over the wrap of second half knot (Fig. 9.3).
- The first half knot will visibly begin to tighten (Fig. 9.4).
- Once adequate level of tightness of first half knot is reached, spill the wrap of second half knot over the tip of assisting instrument (Fig. 9.5).
- Tighten the second half knot (Fig. 9.6).

CORRECTION OF LOOSENING OF FIRST HALF KNOT
- Follow the steps for second half knot
- Tighten without spilling the wraps
- Once adequate tightening is reached, follow the steps of intracorporeal knot tying

UNRAVELING OF KNOT

Factors relating to unraveling of knot include:

- *Incorrect tying technique:* Wrapping around a single thread without crossing, inadequate tightening, loosening and cutting the suture ends too short can give rise to unraveling.
- *Choice of suture material:* Smooth materials like polybutylene and with slippery surface (Gore-tex) are prone to unraveling.

- *Handling of knot:* After tying the knot if only one end is picked, it leads to loosening and can unravel the whole knot.

Remedy

Place another knot in close proximity to the previous knot.

SHORT SUTURE LENGTH ▶

During continuous suturing or during multiple interrupted suturing one may face the trouble of short suture length during intracorporeal knotting. Introducing another suture is an obvious solution, but it increases the traffic of instruments and is time consuming. Tedious frustating attempts at knotting may be wasteful. Following remedy may help if 1-1.5 cm of suture length of the standing part is still available for suturing.

Remedy

Half moon effect

- Short suture length problem (Fig. 9.7) can be curtailed by utilizing the length of the needle for forming the loop. This lengthens the total length available for wrapping (Fig. 9.8).

- The needle is held at short distance from the tip of needle (This is in contrast to the traditional way, in which knotting is done by handling the suture, then the needle). The part of needle towards the suture acts as a prolongation of the suture and can be utilized for forming the loop and subsequent wrapping. Interestingly, the appearance of the needle at this stage looks like a 'half moon' (Figs 9.9 to 9.11).

CAUTION
Handling needle inside abdomen should be done extremely carefully. Inadvertent injury to the viscera can occur at this stage, especially while wrapping and spilling the knots.

HALF MOON EFFECT: MANAGEMENT OF SHORT SUTURE LENGTH

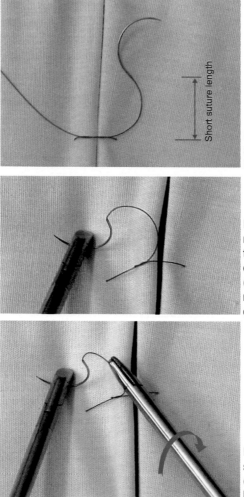

Fig. 9.7: Short suture length available for suturing

Fig. 9.8: Hold the needle and utilize the length of needle for suturing. (Observe the half moon appearance of the needle)

Fig. 9.9: Follow steps of suturing (Wrapping shown here)

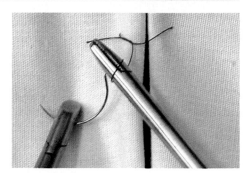

Fig. 9.10: Tail pick-up

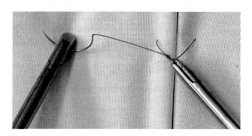

Fig. 9.11: Knot complete

HALF MOON EFFECT: MANAGEMENT OF SHORT SUTURE LENGTH

- Hold the needle near the tip
- Form C loop utilizing the length of needle
- Follow the steps of knot tying

INCORRECT LOOP FORMATION

'S' Loop Formation

If the wrong hand holds the suture then S loop formation can occur which will not result in tying a flat knot (Fig. 9.12).

Reversed 'S' Loop

Again if the suture is held in the wrong hand a reversed S loop can form which will not result in tying a flat knot (Fig. 9.13).

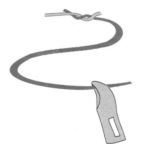 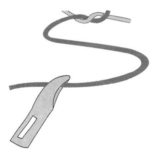

Fig. 9.12: 'S' loop (right instrument instead of left, used for forming 'C' loop for right side)

Fig. 9.13: Reversed 'S' loop (left instrument instead of right used for forming 'C' loop on left side)

'O' Loop

If one tried to tie the knot superior to the stitch, O loop formation may occur, hindering the surgeon's view of the tissues being sutured (Fig. 9.14).

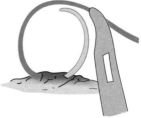

Fig. 9.14: 'O' loop

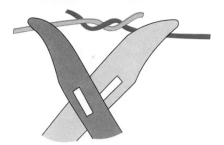

Fig. 9.15: Crossing instruments

CROSSING INSTRUMENTS

Crossing of instruments is clumsy, makes task more time consuming and in doing so the instruments block the view of the surgeon (Fig. 9.15).

NEEDLE DEFLECTION AND REMEDY

A common problem is that when the needle is pushed into the tissue, it will deflect to one side.

Cause

Deviating from the principle of pushing the needle head-on against tissue resistance (Figs 9.16 and 9.17).

Solution

Drive the needle slowly, so that if deflection occurs, the direction of penetration can be corrected (Soft-Grip).

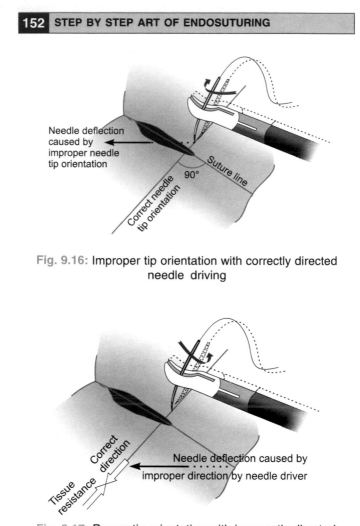

Fig. 9.16: Improper tip orientation with correctly directed
needle driving

Fig. 9.17: Proper tip orientation with incorrectly directed
needle driving

CAUTION

Avoid a rock-solid grip in the attempt to perform suturing as this can cause tearing in the event of inadvertent movement.

COMPLICATIONS OF SUTURING

1. The needle may traumatize the vessel or viscera.

   Remedy
   - Bleeding from injured vessel usually requires nothing more than pressure.
   - Similarly close examination of visceral penetration is all that is needed mostly.

   However potentially fatal injuries are known to occur and one should be extremely cautious in handling intraperitoneal needles.

TIP
- To avoid such injuries, always keep the needle under view.
- Handle the needle by the attached suture except when driving it through the tissues.

2. *Lost needle:* The suture or the needle may be lost intra-abdominally.

   Remedy
   - Always keep the needle under vision to avoid this disturbing complication.

- Tedious radiological localization magnetized probe may be helpful in case of such eventuality.

3. Suture of tissues has the potential to entrap intestine in a ring of tissue. Such a space should be closed.

> *Be near me when my light is low,*
> *when the nerves prick and tingle.*
> *And the heart is sick,*
> *and all the wheels are being slow.*
> —*In memoriam, Tennyson*

Chapter 10

Useful Accessories

- **CLIPS AND CLIP APPLIERS**
- **SEWING DEVICES**
- **LIGATING INSTRUMENTS**
- **ENDOSURGICAL STAPLING**
- **FIBRIN GLUE**
- **BIOFRAGMENTABLE ANASTOMOSIS RING (BAR)**

Everything should be made as simple as possible;
but not more so.

—*Einstein*

CLIPS AND CLIP APPLIERS

Most surgeons are familiar with using the Clip Appliers during laparoscopic cholecystectomy. The traditional **titanium clip** appliers in general, use a 10 mm cannula. A 5 mm clip applier is also available (Ligaclip Allport, Ethicon Endosurgery Inc.) that allows the placement of three 5 mm and one 10 mm port during laparoscopic cholecystectomy, replacing the traditional approach of two 5 mm and two 10 mm ports. Preloaded clip applicator with automatic clip delivery to the jaws has also become available (Endoclip, American AutoStapler). This instrument allows rapid, precise and repeated clipping without the need of withdrawing the instrument to load it, thereby speeding the procedure considerably. Right angle clip appliers are available which enhance visualization of clip appliers back jaw. Non-absorbable metal clips (titanium) are available in various sizes. As in open surgery, selection of the appropriately sized clip for the pedicle in question is important. Care must be taken during their application, and a second clip should be used whenever considered necessary. Traditional titanium clips do have some disadvantages. They have poor lateral grip after application to the pedicle, which can lead to displacement when they are brushed accidentally during manipulations, especially if they are not of the right size in relation to the structure or have not been applied at right angles to its long axis and traction is applied to the clipped structure. They also interfere with both computed tomography and magnetic resonance imaging.

Absorbable polydioxanone clips provide an attractive alternative to metal ones. Applicators designed to allow their laparoscopic use are available. Again, clip selection is important to match the size of the pedicle. If the clip applied is too small or too large, it will not anchor securely and will tend to slip off the pedicle. Absorption of these clips takes about 6 months.

> **CAUTION**
> Some surgeons use clips on the end of sutures instead of knots. Whilst undoubtedly quicker, this practice is unsafe as the grip on the suture material by the clip is not secure enough, and it comes off easily with the minimum of traction.

The only clip which is strong enough to hold the suture is made of silver **(Silver Beads)** and this is used in endoluminal rectal surgery. Resorbable clips with similar grip strength are being developed.

The **ligature clip** produced by origin works on the principles of the ligature clips of open surgery. The arc-shaped clip captures the pedicle when its tips come in contact prior to full closure. The rectangular, hook-like orientation of the clips and applier provides improved control of the actual clipping process.

A new absorbable **lapro clip** consisting of two parts has been introduced by Davis and Geek (Wayne, NJ, JSA). The relatively elastic inner member (polygly-conate) is approximated prior to full closure so that the pedicle can be grasped. Subsequently, the rigid outer member (polygycolic acid) is pushed over the inner member and thus the clip completely and firmly locked. Each clip is mounted into a complete tip of the forceps, which is disposable, whereas handle and shaft are reusable parts.

The new **Hem-lock-clip** by Linvatec Weck (Largo, FL, USA) shows some principal improvements. The locking ends provide excellent tissue penetration and the fixation at the tissue is improved due to the concave-convex shape of the branches. This clip is nonabsorbable, which lowers its value. Further testing of these clips is necessary before final clinical application. As all metals more or less interfere with imaging procedures such as CT and MRI, clips made from synthetic material are preferable.

Clips for tissue approximation include the 10 mm **endohernia multiple staplers** whose U-shaped clip is deformed to a close square. Although their efficacy in endoscopic hernia repair with mesh has been proven, the long-term effects caused by these clips to the surrounding tissue are unclear. Another alternative is the **Tack Applier** (Origin Medical, Menlo Park, CA) which consist of corkscrew tacks for securing a mesh during laparoscopic hernia repair and has the advantage of insertion through a 5 mm cannula.

SEWING DEVICES

The requirements of an endoscopic sewing device are that it is reliable, fast, safe and provides easy tissue approximation with atraumatic needle and thread design. The needle should be easily held and one should be able to stitch in various directions with various knotting techniques at reasonable cost per procedure. The device should be easily maintained and cleaned if it has reusable parts.

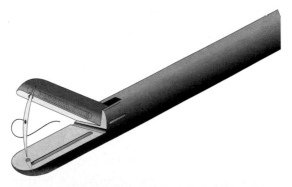

Fig. 10.1: Endostitch, US Surgical Corporation

A needle with two pointed trocars with a central cross-bore as thread housing was introduced many years ago to surgery. However, the shuttle needle requires transfer between two needle drivers. A breakthrough for the management of needle and thread is achieved by shuttling the needle between the jaws of the same instrument. One such disposable product (**Endostitch**, US Surgical Corporation) (Fig. 10.1) has been available since 1994. This 10 mm instrument is equipped with double action jaws each of which has a gripping system for the needle which is operated by an attached lever at the axial handle. These gripping elements are simple stainless steel bands which fit into cross-sectional grooves pressed into the needle proximal to the trocar point. This instrument has been shown to reduce the time needed for the placement of stitches and knot tying.

LIGATING INSTRUMENTS

The execution of a ligature with thread requires delicate handling with two forceps to pass the tie around the vessel and the creation of an external slip knot. Although the tie can be appropriately passed using curved instruments, the development of instruments especially for ligature is important.

The passage of the thread around a vessel can be facilitated using superelastic material, e.g. **Nitinol**. The thread is passed with a superelastic wire surround the pedicle. Nitinol wire, which features stress-induced martensitie phase transformation, can be preshaped using special heat treatment. It can then be introduced in a restraining tube. When extruded it recovers its pre-formed curved shape. Thread can be inserted through a needle eye at the distal end and then passed around a pedicle. The thread is subsequently grasped by a forceps and the ligature then finished with an external slip knot or a knot clip.

ENDOSURGICAL STAPLING

Surgical stapling systems were developed and used for decades in eastern Europe and the Soviet Union. Later, they were introduced in the United States. The ancients used ants to close wounds, which is probably the inspiration for the Von Petz and later surgical staplers. The history of stapler development began in the early 1900s and continues today. The laparoscopic 30 mm linear stapling and cutting device was first introduced in the United States in 1990.

The development of this endoscopic instrument had to overcome many obstacles, including the need to decrease the size of the instrumentation to fit available cannulae, operation of the stapler remote from the handle, availability of interchangeable cartridges with varying staple size, ability to operate the instrument with one hand, ability to ligate small and big vessels, and the need for rotary articulation of the stapler to apply staples at appropriate angles. Successful co-operation between clinicians and biomedical engineers produced the linear stapler and cutting devices. The staples vary in size depending on whether vascular or non-vascular tissue is being transacted. Vascular staplers compress to 1 mm and non-vascular staples compress to 1.5 mm on firing. The 30 mm linear stapler and cutting device needs to be placed through a 12 mm cannula. There are 45 and 60 mm staplers in the market that are placed through a 12 and 18 mm cannulae respectively.

The nature of most laparoscopic instruments requires a length adequate to reach through the cannula to within the abdomen. Once the jaw of the linear stapler and cutting device is closed the instrument may be used as a lever to manipulate the tissues. Unnecessary tissue trauma can be caused by injudicious use of such force. It is at times difficult to visualize the most distal portion because of the length of the stapler, but this is vital to ensure that it is free of underlying vital structures; an angled laparoscope is valuable in this regard. The 30 mm linear stapler and cutting device can be used during laparoscopic appendicectomy to staple across the base of the appendix and meso-appendix, or to fashion a side to side anastomosis.

Staplers have been found to shorten operative procedure times and thus result in cost savings although this may not be true for all surgical applications. When compared with bipolar coagulation and ligature placement in performing laparoscopic oopherectomy there was found to be no differences in operative time, hospital admission rates or complications among the three groups. A new linear stapler and cutting device has been developed with the ability to articulate the angle of the stapler. Such a modification may improve the ability to reach difficult areas without placing an additional cannula.

FIBRIN GLUE

Hemostasis has been achieved using fibrin glue in hepatic and splenic lacerations, in partial nephrectomy and for sealing vascular anastomoses. The use of fibrin tissue adhesives has been proposed in many surgical disciplines. Fibrin glue has been used for laparoscopic ureteral resection and anastomosis, to control hemorrhage via diagnostic laparoscopy for splenic trauma, laparoscopic repair of perforated peptic ulcer, and laparoscopic choledochojejunostomy. Fibrin glue may offer promise in the future to assist with anastomosis, tissue approximation and hemostasis.

BIOFRAGMENTABLE ANASTOMOSIS RING (BAR)

This device was introduced in 1985 and is similar to the original metal Murphy's button which was first described in 1892. The BAR is a double segmented ring originally designed for colonic anastomosis and is constructed of polyglycolic acid impregnated with barium sulphate. The bowel segment to be anastomosed are anchored with purse string sutures after which the halves are compressed digitally. A circumferential serosa to serosa contact is formed with even compression without any tissue piercing material at the anastomotic line.

The ring fragments in about 3 weeks and the pieces are expelled with the feces. This method has proved its value in several trials of colonic surgery as well as for small bowel anastomosis. In addition this device has been used to perform laparoscopic intestinal surgery in an animal model and has also been reported to laparoscopic assisted left hemicolectomy. This technology might be useful in helping to perform anastomosis if the device can be altered for laparoscopic use.

Although devices are commercially available to facilitate certain suturing scenarios, we believe that none of the operations can be completed as effectively by using a suture device then to sew manually. The ability to suture laparoscopically markedly broadens the number of clinical scenarios in which minimal access techniques can be used.

Chapter 11

The Future…
is Here!

Belief in truth begins with doubting all that has hitherto been believed to be true.

—*Nietzche*

Much research has been done on the value of three dimensional vision systems, which may improve laparoscopic suturing by less experienced surgeons.

Telemanipulation and telepresence is a field that is being applied to perform complex human tasks either within remote areas, such as outer space or deep beneath the ocean, or inaccessible and inhospitable fields, such as radioactive and biologically contaminated areas.

Work is in progress in the development of robots that can perform the fine suturing required during endoscopic coronary artery bypass surgery. The Zeus robot (Computer Motion Inc., Goleta, CA), a robotic enhancement device designed to perform and fine tune the movements made by human hands, might be useful for minimally invasive cardiac surgery and possibly other roles in laparoscopic surgery in the near future. The surgeon uses hand grips and foot pedals on the console to control three robotic arms that perform the surgery using a variety of surgical tools. The product, the Da Vinci Surgical System, made by Intuitive Surgical, Inc., of Mountain View, Calif., is the first of its kind. The robotic arms, which have a "wrist" built in to the end of the tool, give surgeons additional manipulation ability during laparoscopic surgery, enabling easier, more intricate motion and better control of surgical tools.

Laparoscopic surgery is evolving and its applications are growing to include most abdominal operations. Tissue approximation by means other than mechanical clips or staples is becoming increasingly important. Today's surgeon is driven by the desire to perform a given procedure under laparoscopic guidance as well as, if not better than, under laparotomy. The ability to suture laparoscopically and to use all the stapling techniques available greatly adds to the level of comfort and confidence of the endoscope surgeon. If surgeons do not feel comfortable with laparoscopic suturing, they should question whether or not the procedure should be performed endoscopically.

"No future without suture."!

Index

A

Aberdeen knot, 86
Amount of bite, 65
Angle
    azimuth, 20
    elevation, 20
    manipulation, 20, 43
    needle holding, 44
    needle insertion, 44
Appendiceal mesentery ligation,
    7
Azimuth angles, 20

B

Bioframentable anastomosis
    ring (BAR), 163
Bite
    amount, 65
    entrance, 65
    exit, 65

C

Castroviejo needle holder, 34
Choledochotomy closure, 10
Chopstick effect, 43
Choreography-of-movements
    technique, 21, 88
Coaxial handle design, 37
Complications of suturing,153
    remedy, 153
Continuous suturing, 72
Cook needle holder, 34, 35

'C' loop creation, 90, 93
Clips
    polydioxanone, 157
    titanium, 156
Crossing instruments, 151
Curved needle, 28, 29

D

Dorsey bowel grasper, 76
Driving the needle, 62
Ductal anastomosis, 74
Duncan slip knot, 137

E

Elevation angle, 20
End to end suturing, 75
End to side suturing, 75
Endoclip, 156
Endohernia stapler, 158
Endoloop, 30
Endoscope-to-target distance, 20
Endoscopic gastrointestinal
    anastomosis (GIA)
    stapler, 161
Endostitch, 160
Entrance point, 65
Ergonomics in intracorporeal
    suturing, 21, 108
Ethicon needle holder, 35
Exit bite, 65
Extracorporeal knotting, 110
    advantages, 111
    drawbacks, 140

F

Fibrin glue, 163
First assistant, 20
Fisherman's knot, 137

G

GIA stapler, 161
Grasping forceps, 39

H

Half moon effect, 146-149
Hand instruments, 31
Hand-eye-co-ordination, 17
Handle design
    coaxial, 37
    pistol type, 37
Hem-lock-clip, 158
Hiatal hernia, 10
Horizontal suturing, 42

I

Ideal knot, 81
Indian rope trick, 139
Instrumentation, 25
Interrupted suturing, 71
Intracorporeal knotting, 79
    advantages, 81
    technique, 88-101
Intracorporeal suturing, 69
Intracorporeal twist technique,
    101
Intracorporeal-extracorporeal
    ratio, 44

J

Jamming slip knot, 84

K

Knot
    extracorporeal, 113
    intracorporeal, 81
    ligature slip, 83
    loosening of, 142
    square slip, 82, 103-107
    square, 81
    substitutes, 107
    surgeon's, 84
    tayside, 137, 138
    Texas endosurgery, 135, 136
    unraveling of, 145
Knot pushers
    metal, 39
    plastic, 39
Knot substitutes, 107

L

Laparoscopic appendectomy, 10
Laparoscopic cholecystectomy,
    10, 15
Lapo Tract M.I.S. support
    system, 20
Lapraty knot clip, 107
Lapro clip, 158
Lapromed, 37
Ligation in continuity, 111
Ligature clip, 157
Ligature slip knot, 83
Linear incisions closure, 71
Loading needle, 55
Loosening of knot, 142
    correction of loosening, 142-45
    factors associated, 142

M

Manipulation angle, 20, 43
Melzer knot, 124-135

Metal knot pusher, 39
Micro-surgery, 15, 18
Motor skill, 18

N

Natural positioning, 42
Needle
    adjustment of, 55
    curved, 28
    loading, 55
    ski, 28
    straight, 28
Needle deflection, 151
    remedy, 151
Needle holder
    Cook, 34, 35
    Ethicon, 35
    MBG, 35, 36
    Self-righting, 37
    Semm, 32
    Szabo-Berci, 36
    Wolfe, 34, 35
Needle holding angle, 45
Needle introduction, 45
    percutaneous, 51
    using 5 mm reducer, 45–51
    using 5 mm port, 51
    using 10 mm port, 52
Nitinol, 160

O

'O' loop, 150
Offset positioning, 42

P

Pistol type handles, 37
Plastic knot pusher, 39
Polydioxanone clips, 157
Port placement, 43

Positioning
    natural, 42
    offset, 42
Prerequisite for suturing, 16

R

Reich method, 51
Reversed 'S' loop, 150
Roeder knot 100, 114-123

S

'S' loop, 150
Self-righting needle holder, 37
Semm needle holder, 32
Sense of feel, 13
Sewing device, 159
Short suture length, 140
    remedy, 146
Side to side anastomosis, 75
Silver beads, 157
Ski-shaped needle, 28
Square knot, 81
Square slip knot, 82, 103-107
    advantages, 82
Straight needle, 28
Suturing
    continuous, 72
    horizontal, 42
    interrupted, 71
    vertical, 42
Surgeon's knot, 84
Surgitie, 30
Sword fighting, 14
Szabo-Berci needle holders, 36

T

Tack applier, 159
Tail pick up, 91, 96
Tayside knot, 137, 138

Telemanipulation, 166
Telepresence surgery, 166
Texas Endosurgery Institute
    knot, 135
Tissue handling, 21
Titanium clip, 156
Training, 22

U

Unraveling of knot
    factors associated, 145
    remedy, 146
Utility of laparoscopic suturing,
    10

V

Vascular stapler, 162
Vertical suturing, 42
Visual perception–eye-hand
    coordination, 17

W

Wolfe needle holder, 34, 35
Wrapping, 90, 94

Z

Zeus robot, 166